O A I D L
OXFORD AMERICAN INFECTIOUS DISEASE LIBRARY

Hepatitis C

O A I D L

OXFORD AMERICAN INFECTIOUS DISEASE LIBRARY

Hepatitis C

Donald Jensen

Professor of Medicine; Director, Center for Liver Disease
University of Chicago Medical Center
Chicago, IL

Nancy Reau

Associate Professor of Medicine, Center for Liver Disease
University of Chicago Medical Center
Chicago, IL

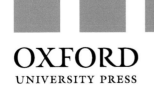

OXFORD
UNIVERSITY PRESS

OXFORD

UNIVERSITY PRESS

Oxford University Press is a department of the University of Oxford.
It furthers the University's objective of excellence in research, scholarship,
and education by publishing worldwide.

Oxford   New York
Auckland   Cape Town   Dar es Salaam   Hong Kong   Karachi
Kuala Lumpur   Madrid   Melbourne   Mexico City   Nairobi
New Delhi   Shanghai   Taipei   Toronto

With offices in
Argentina   Austria   Brazil   Chile   Czech Republic   France   Greece
Guatemala   Hungary   Italy   Japan   Poland   Portugal   Singapore
South Korea   Switzerland   Thailand   Turkey   Ukraine   Vietnam

Oxford is a registered trademark of Oxford University Press in the UK
and certain other countries.

Published in the United States of America by
Oxford University Press
198 Madison Avenue, New York, NY 10016

© Oxford University Press 2013

Library of Congress Cataloging-in-Publication Data

Hepatitis C / [edited by] Donald Jensen, Nancy Reau.
p. ; cm. — (Oxford American infectious disease library)
Includes bibliographical references.
ISBN 978-0-19-984429-6 (pbk. : alk. paper)
I. Jensen, Donald.   II. Reau, Nancy.   III. Series: Oxford American infectious disease library.
[DNLM: 1. Hepatitis C. WC 536]
616.3'623—dc23
2012011003

1 3 5 7 9 8 6 4 2
Printed in the United States of America
on acid-free paper

Disclosures

Andres F. Carrion has nothing to disclose.

Stanley Martin Cohen has been on speakers bureaus from Bristol-Meyers Squibb, Gilead, Genentech, and Vertex; on advisory boards for BMS, Gilead, and Vertex; and a consultant for BMS and Gilead.

Leslie Dawvaroo has nothing to disclose.

Archita P. Desai has nothing to disclose.

Michael W. Fried has received research grants from Genentech, Merck, Vertex, Tibotec, Gilead, Bristol-Meyers Squibb, Anadys, Contaus, and Abbott; has been a consultant for Genentech, Tibotech, Vertex, Merck Pharmasset, Glaxo, Novartis, Abbott, and Gilead; and has received research grants from the NIH.

Christin M. Giordano has nothing to disclose.

Shriram Jakate has nothing to disclose.

Donald M. Jensen is on the Consulting and Advisory Boards for Abbott, Boehringer-Ingelheim, Genentech/Roche, Johnson & Johnson/Tibotec, Merck, Pharmasset/Gilead, Vertex; has received research grants from Abbott, Boehringer-Ingelheim, Genentech/Roche, Johnson & Johnson/ Tibotec, Merck, Pharmasset/Gilead, Vertex; has spoken at Consensus Medical Communications, Projects in Knowledge, Clinical Care Options; and has had a publication for SLACK, Inc.

Leila Kia has nothing to disclose.

Arthur Y. Kim has served as consultant to Vertex Pharmaceuticals and has received research funding from the National Institutes of Health (NIAID and NIDA).

Josh Levitsky is on the Speaker Bureau for Genentech and Vertex.

Paul Martin served as a consultant for Vertex, Genetech, Abbott, and Merck.

Kristina A. Matkowskyj has nothing to disclose.

Christopher E. McGowan has nothing to disclose.

Anjana A. Pillai is a speaker for Merck and Otsuka.

Nancy Reau has served on the advisory boards of BMS, Vertex, Gilead, and Genetech/Roche and as a consultant to Merck. She has received research support from Vertex and Gilead.

Dedication

We dedicate this book to our family, friends, colleagues, and trainees who have inspired, motivated, and encouraged us during its preparation.

Preface

Rapid and profound changes are taking place in the field of hepatitis C therapeutics. Within the next few years we may be able to cure more than 90% of infected patients who seek treatment, and an interferon-free therapy is a realistic possibility. More than ever, these rapid therapeutic changes compel us to review the broader scope of hepatitis C, including its epidemiology, diagnostics, natural history, and clinical features. Given the accelerated advance in hepatitis C knowledge, a review of these features requires a shortened timeline from concept to publication. Our goal in the preparation of this handbook is to provide the fundamentals of our knowledge of hepatitis C to allow readers to quickly survey the field, yet with the confidence that the information is current and accurate.

The first five chapters provide the framework for the more clinical chapters to come. Randall describes in clear and understandable terms the basic biology of the hepatitis C virus in Chapter 1. It is this information that has led to the development of direct-acting antiviral agents and is thus essential reading. In Chapter 2 Te discusses the epidemiology of hepatitis C, including the geographic prevalence of the various HCV genotypes—an important consideration given globalization and international travel. In Chapter 3 Jenkins and Aronsohn discuss the natural history of HCV, including current information regarding risk factors for transmission. Diagnostic testing for HCV is presented by Walzer and Cotler in Chapter 4, which includes a concise overview of nucleic acid testing limitations and use. In Chapter 5, Jakate details the histopathologic features of acute and chronic HCV infection and the importance of the grading scale used to define inflammatory and fibrosis components. These first five chapters represent the key background information on which most clinical decision making is based.

The relatively uncommon but important issue of acute hepatitis C is discussed by Price and Kim in Chapter 6, including the serologic diagnosis. Satoskar discusses chronic hepatitis C in Chapter 7, providing an overview and recapitulation of its natural history. The importance and evaluation of the extrahepatic manifestations of chronic hepatitis C are elaborated by Robertazzi and Pillai in Chapter 8. This is followed by a thorough review of the issues facing liver transplantation consideration in HCV subjects, as nicely outlined by Kia, Matkowskyj, and Levitsky in Chapter 9.

The remaining chapters focus on HCV treatment. An overview of treatment candidacy and current considerations is presented by Dawravoo and Cohen in Chapter 10. This is followed in Chapter 11 by an important review of side effect management by McGowan and Fried, focusing on those events attributable to peginterferon and ribavirin. In Chapter 12 Carrion, Giordano, and Martin present a case-based approach to HCV treatment in special populations, including those with chronic kidney disease, those who have undergone liver transplant, and those with HIV co-infection. Poordad discusses the current genotype 1 standard of care with telaprevir and boceprevir in Chapter 13, which sets the stage for a further discussion of newer direct-acting antivirals in clinical development by Ahn and Flamm in Chapter 14. Finally, Desai and Reau provide a useful review of the lexicon of the numerous clinical trials in HCV drug development in Chapter 15.

We hope that readers will find this book both informative and clinically useful. We have attempted to keep verbiage to a minimum while presenting key points in easily referenced tables. In a rapidly moving field, this book offers the reader a valuable pocket resource for years to come.

Nancy Reau, MD
Donald Jensen, MD

Contents

Contributors

Joseph Ahn, MD, MS
Assistant Professor of Medicine
Loyola University Medical Center
Maywood, IL

Andrew Aronsohn, MD
Assistant Professor of Medicine
University of Chicago
Chicago, IL

Andres F. Carrion, MD
Division of Gastroenterology
University of Miami Miller School
of Medicine
Miami, FL

Stanley Martin Cohen, MD
Associate Professor, Medicine,
Gastroenterology, Hepatology &
Nutrition
Director, Section of Hepatology
Loyola University Medical Center
Maywood, IL

Scott Cotler, MD
Associate Professor of Medicine
Chief, Section of Hepatology
University of Illinois Medical
Center
Chicago, IL

Lesley Dawravoo, MD
Gastroenterology Fellow
Loyola University Medical Center
Maywood, IL

Archita P. Desai, MD
Department of Internal Medicine
University of Chicago
Chicago, IL

Steven L. Flamm, MD
Professor of Medicine
Northwestern Feinberg School of
Medicine
Chicago, IL

Michael W. Fried, MD
UNC Liver Center
University of North Carolina at
Chapel Hill
Chapel Hill, NC

**Christin M. Giordano, MPAS,
PA-C**
Division of Hepatology
University of Miami Miller School
of Medicine
Miami, FL

Shriram Jakate, MD, FRCPath
Professor of Pathology,
Gastroenterology and Hepatology
Rush University Medical Center
Chicago, IL

Erin Jenkins, MD
Fellow, Department of
Gastroenterology, Hepatology, and
Nutrition
University of Chicago
Chicago, IL

Leila Kia, MD
Deparment of Internal Medicine
Northwestern University, Feinberg
School of Medicine.
Chicago, IL

Arthur Y. Kim, MD
Assistant Professor of Medicine
Division of Infectious Diseases
Massachusetts General Hospital
Harvard Medical School
Boston, MA

Josh Levitsky, MD, MS
Associate Professor in Medicine-
Gastroenterology and Hepatology
and Surgery-Organ Transplantation
Comprehensive Transplant Center
Northwestern University Feinberg
School of Medicine
Chicago, IL

Paul Martin, MD
Division of Hepatology
University of Miami Miller School
of Medicine
Miami, FL

**Kristina A. Matkowskyj, MD,
PhD**
Fellow, Department of Pathology
Northwestern University Feinberg
School of Medicine
Chicago, IL

Christopher E. McGowan, MD
UNC Liver Center
University of North Carolina at
Chapel Hill
Chapel Hill, NC

Anjana A. Pillai, MD
Division of Gastroenterology,
Hepatology and Nutrition
Loyola University Medical Center
Maywood, IL

Fred Poordad, MD
Associate Professor of Medicine
David Geffen School of
Medicine at UCLA
Chief, Hepatology and Liver
Transplantation
Cedars-Sinai Medical Center
Los Angeles, CA

Christin N. Price, MD
Department of Medicine
Brigham and Women's Hospital
Harvard Medical School
Boston, MA

Glenn Randall, PhD
Assistant Professor, Department of
Microbiology
Biological Sciences Division
University of Chicago
Chicago, IL

Nancy Reau, MD
Associate Professor of Medicine,
Center for Liver Disease
University of Chicago Medical
Center
Chicago, IL

Suzanne Robertazzi, ANP
Division of Gastroenterology,
Hepatology and Nutrition
Loyola University Medical Center
Maywood, IL

Rohit Satoskar, MD
Assistant Professor of Medicine
and Surgery, Georgetown
Transplant Institute
Georgetown University Hospital
Washington, DC

Helen S. Te, MD
Associate Professor of Medicine
Medical Director of Liver
Transplantation
Center for Liver Diseases
University of Chicago Medical
Center
Chicago, Illinois

Natasha Walzer, MD
Instructor of Medicine,
Department of Hepatology
University of Illinois College of
Medicine at Chicago
Chicago, IL

Chapter 1

Basic Virology

Glenn Randall

The Virus

The structure of hepatitis C virus (HCV), called a virion, is shown in Figure 1.1. Unlike humans, the genetic material of HCV is ribonucleic acid (RNA). The genome is one long RNA strand containing ~9,600 nucleotides (Moradpour et al., 2007). The RNA is protected from the environment by a protein shell called a capsid. Surrounding the capsid is a lipid membrane called an envelope. The envelope is acquired from human membranes and contains the viral envelope proteins, E1 and E2. The envelope proteins bind receptor proteins on human liver cells to initiate infection. The size of the HCV virions vary, but they are ~ 60 nanometers in diameter. One reason that it is difficult to develop antiviral drugs, as opposed to antibiotics that target bacteria, is that the viral envelope is covered in our own membrane and thus is not chemically distinct from our own cells. Bacterial cell walls are chemically different and can be targeted by drugs like penicillin.

Viruses are simple genetically and do not contain all of the information they need to replicate. Instead, they depend on target cells to perform some of the key functions in the viral life cycle. For instance, viruses are not capable of producing proteins since they do not contain ribosomes. Instead they use cellular ribosomes to make their proteins. This is another reason why antiviral drugs are difficult to develop, as opposed to antibiotics. Bacteria have their own protein synthesis machinery that is different from ours that can be specifically targeted. Since viruses use many cellular functions it is more difficult to selectively target them without harming the patient.

HCV Quasispecies and Genotypes

There is a great amount of variation in the RNA sequences of HCV genomes, shown in Figure 1.2. This is due in part to its mode of replication. DNA genetic information is relatively stable because the enzymes that synthesize DNA, called DNA polymerases, have proofreading activity: They can recognize mistakes in the DNA sequence and edit them. RNA genomes are more variable because RNA polymerases lack proofreading activity. The HCV RNA polymerase makes a mistake once every 10,000 nucleotides, which coincidentally is about the size of its genome. Thus, each new viral genome contains approximately

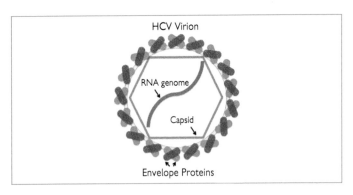

Figure 1.1 The HCV virion

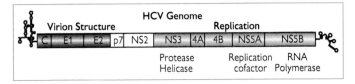

Figure 1.2 The HCV genome

one different base from its parent virus. These mutations can be either detrimental to the virus by disrupting an essential viral function, neutral, or in some cases beneficial, as described below.

A chronically infected individual produces ~10^{12} HCV genomes every day, most of which vary slightly from each other due to these RNA polymerase mistakes (Neumann et al., 1998). Collectively, these variant viruses within the same infected person are called quasispecies. HCV quasispecies present a formidable challenge to treating infection. Although the virus variants are similar to each other, sometimes the small differences can have a major impact on a virus evading the immune system or developing drug resistance. Our adaptive immune responses to HCV (1) produce antibodies that bind HCV virions to prevent infection and (2) activate T-cell responses, which kill infected cells that are presenting parts of viral proteins on their surface. These immune responses typically target the most abundant virus variants and are effective at eliminating them. However, rare HCV variants that contain mutations in the parts of the proteins that are recognized by the immune responses have changed enough that they can escape control by the immune system. These variants become dominant in the infected person until they, in turn, are eventually recognized and subsequently targeted by immune cells. Then another HCV variant that is resistant to the immune response emerges. This evolutionary "arms race" between the virus and the immune system is a hallmark of chronic viral infections.

Quasispecies are also a problem with antiviral drug resistance. Minor HCV variants that are resistant to a drug can be selected to emerge and become dominant just as above. This is the reason why single drugs cannot be used to effectively treat HIV or HCV. It is too easy for drug resistance to emerge. However, when drugs that target different viral proteins or functions are combined, then resistance is less likely to emerge. It is mathematically less likely for a virus to acquire all of the mutations to become resistant to multiple drugs.

As HCV has evolved in the population, the variations in genome sequences have become more dramatic. HCV has been classified into six genotypes, which vary from each other by over 30% at the nucleotide level (Simmonds et al., 2005). Viruses within the same genotype are more similar in sequence to each other than they are to an HCV isolate from a different genotype. These genotypes are thought to largely reflect the geographical distribution of the virus. Genotype 1 is the predominant genotype in the Americas, Europe, and Northern Asia and thus is the primary focus of drug development. The virus genotype can also affect the response to therapy. Patients who are infected with genotypes 1 and 4 respond to interferon-plus-ribavirin therapy only 40% to 50% of the time, while those with genotype 2 and 3 respond 80% to 90% of the time (Hnatyszyn, 2005; Steinkuhler et al., 1996). Thus, the genotype of the virus is an important criterion when evaluating whether a patient should undergo interferon-plus-ribavirin therapy. There are also genotype-specific differences in the response to the newly developed drugs that directly target viral proteins. These responses vary depending on the drug, but most drugs are biased to be more effective against genotype 1, since it is the predominant HCV genotype in developed countries.

HCV Replication and Drug Targets

HCV completes its life cycle in a liver cell, shown in Figure 1.3, in approximately one day. It first infects liver cells by directly engaging a series of cellular proteins, called receptors, which are expressed on the outside surface of liver cells. The virion enters the liver cell following engagement of the receptors and is delivered to enclosed compartments called endosomes. When the endosomes reach an acidic pH, the virion envelope fuses with the endosomal membrane and the virion uncoats, delivering its RNA genome into the cytoplasm of cells. The beginning of the viral genome contains an RNA structure that directly binds human ribosomes, which initiates the translation of the HCV genome into one long protein. This long protein is then cut into at least 10 individual proteins by enzymes called proteases. The long HCV protein is cut by cellular and viral proteases. The viral NS3 protease cleaves the replication proteins (Steinkuhler et al., 1996) and is a critical target for new HCV drugs. These drugs typically bind NS3 near its active site and prevent its ability to cut the long HCV protein into individual proteins (De Francesco et al., 1999). Without protease cleavage, HCV is unable to replicate. May 2011 marked a milestone for HCV therapy when the first two drugs targeting a HCV protein, in this case the NS3 protease, received approval from the U.S. Food and Drug Administration.

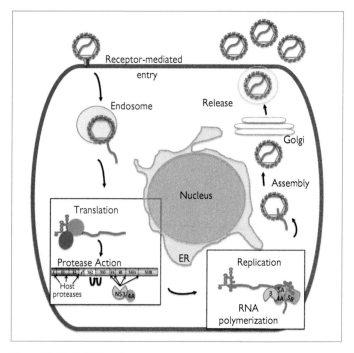

Figure 1.3 The HCV life cycle

Once the individual proteins are produced, viral replication can initiate. The viral proteins NS3, NS4A, NS4B, NS5A, and NS5B form the replication complex. NS5B performs a critical function in replication: it is the RNA-dependent RNA polymerase. This means that it uses RNA as a template to synthesize new RNA. HCV replicates through a double-stranded RNA intermediate. The replication complex binds to the end of the HCV genome and then NS5B synthesizes a complementary RNA. The complementary RNA can then in turn be used to serve as a template for the synthesis of HCV genomic RNAs. These genomic RNAs can be either translated to make more HCV proteins or assembled into virions. These virions then leave the cell by the secretory pathway and are released from the cell to initiate infection of a new cell.

The activity of the NS5B polymerase is the second major target of new HCV drugs. There are different ways to inhibit polymerases. The first class of drugs are called nucleoside analogues. These resemble RNA nucleosides that are phosphorylated and then incorporated into the newly viral RNA, but they lack chemical features that are required for linking new nucleotides to it. Thus, the elongating RNA is stopped, a process referred to as *chain termination*. A second mechanism of polymerase inhibition is nucleoside-like drugs that compete with real nucleotides for binding to the polymerase. Finally, some drugs bind the polymerase outside of its active site and alter the structure of the polymerase so that it no longer functions (De Francesco & Migliaccio, 2005).

There are some HCV drugs that work in ways we do not currently understand. Screening chemical libraries for compounds that inhibit HCV replication or virus production identified most of the drugs in this category. One such drug works at very low concentrations and is thought to target NS5A because mutations that produce resistance to the drug map to NS5A (Gao et al., 2010). Other potential drugs in early stages of development target the viral entry process or cellular proteins that are required for viral replication (Vermehren & Sarrazin, 2011). As is the case with HIV antivirals, it is anticipated that all stages of the viral life cycle contain legitimate targets for antiviral intervention. We expect that the list of HCV drug targets will continue to expand.

References

De Francesco, R., & G. Migliaccio. (2005). Challenges and successes in developing new therapies for hepatitis C. *Nature, 436*(7053), 953–960.

De Francesco, R., A. Pessi, & C. Steinkuhler. (1999). Mechanisms of hepatitis C virus NS3 proteinase inhibitors. *J Viral Hepat, 6*(Suppl 1), 23–30.

Gao, M., et al. (2010). Chemical genetics strategy identifies an HCV NS5A inhibitor with a potent clinical effect. *Nature, 465*(7294), 96–100.

Hnatyszyn, H. J. (2005). Chronic hepatitis C and genotyping: the clinical significance of determining HCV genotypes. *Antivir Ther, 10*(1), 1–11.

Moradpour, D., F. Penin, & C. M. Rice. (2007). Replication of hepatitis C virus. *Nat Rev Microbiol, 5*(6), 453–463.

Neumann, A. U., et al. (1998). Hepatitis C viral dynamics in vivo and the antiviral efficacy of interferon-alpha therapy. *Science, 282*(5386), 103–107.

Simmonds, P., et al. (2005). Consensus proposals for a unified system of nomenclature of hepatitis C virus genotypes. *Hepatology, 42*(4), 962–973.

Steinkuhler, C., et al. (1996). Activity of purified hepatitis C virus protease NS3 on peptide substrates. *J Virol, 70*(10), 6694–6700.

Vermehren, J., & C. Sarrazin. (2011). New HCV therapies on the horizon. *Clin Microbiol Infect, 17*(2), 122–134.

Chapter 2

Epidemiology of Hepatitis C

Helen S. Te

Introduction

Hepatitis C is an RNA virus known to infect humans and chimpanzees, causing a similar disease in these two species. It is the most common cause of transfusion-related hepatitis and is one of the leading causes of end-stage liver disease requiring liver transplantation in the United States. It is transmitted most efficiently by parenteral means, particularly with large or repeated exposure to infected blood products or transplantation of infected tissue or organ grafts, and intravenous drug use. Less frequently, it can be transmitted by mucosal exposures to blood or serum-derived fluids through perinatal or sexual means (Recommendations for prevention and control, 1998).

The relative mutability of its genome has been blamed for its high propensity to cause chronic infection. About 80% of new infections progress on to chronic infection, with cirrhosis developing in about 20% of infected individuals after 20 to 30 years, resulting in increased risk for liver-related complications and hepatocellular carcinoma (HCC). The high mutability of the HCV genome and limited knowledge of the protective immune response following infection has hindered progress in vaccine development. For this reason, no vaccine is available against HCV (WHO, 2000).

Worldwide Prevalence and Disease Burden

The WHO estimated global prevalence of HCV infection was 3%, or 170 million individuals, in 1999. The prevalence was higher in some countries in Africa (5.3%, or 31.9 million), the Eastern Mediterranean (4.6%, or 21.3 million), Southeast Asia (2.15%, or 32.3 million), and the Western Pacific (3.9%, or 62.2 million) as compared to some countries in the Americas (1.7%, or 13.1 million) and Europe (1.03%, or 8.9 million) (WHO, 2000). In 2004, the Global Burden of Hepatitis C Working Group, serving as a consultant to WHO, estimated the global prevalence to be slightly lower at 2.2%, or 130 million individuals. The lowest HCV prevalence of 0.01% to 0.1% is from countries in the United Kingdom and Scandinavia, while the highest prevalence of 15% to 20% is from Egypt (Alter, 2007) (Fig. 2.1). Hepatitis C is estimated to be the cause of 27% of cirrhosis cases and 25% of HCC cases worldwide (Perz et al., 2006).

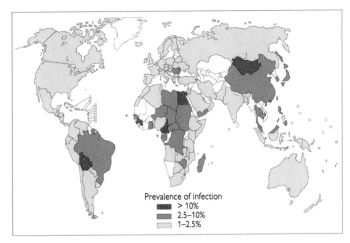

Figure 2.1 Geographic distribution of hepatitis C infection worldwide. (Data from Center for Disease Prevention. Yellow Book 2012 Edition. Available at: http://wwwnc. cdc.gov/travel/yellowbook/2012/chapter-3-infectious-diseases-related-to-travel/hepatitis-c.htm. Accessed April 30, 2012)

High prevalences of HCV of >70% have been reported in injecting drug users and in hemophiliacs, while prevalences of 20% to 30% have been observed in patients on hemodialysis (van der Poel, 1999). The incidence of acute infection is declining since screening of blood products and universal precautions in medical settings have been instituted, with most cases being due to high-risk injection practices (EASL, 1999). However, the prevalence of complications from chronic infection such as cirrhosis and HCC is increasing with time as the infected population group ages. HCV is estimated to cause 8,000 to 10,000 deaths per year related to liver complications and HCC (Alter, 2007).

Genotypes

There are 11 HCV genotypes (genotype 1 to 11), many subtypes (a, b, c, etc.), and about 100 different strains (1, 2, 3, etc.) based on the sequence heterogeneity of the HCV genome. Genotypes 1 to 3 are widely distributed globally, with genotypes 1a and 1b accounting for 60% of infections worldwide (Fig. 2.2). Genotype 1a is predominantly located in Northern Europe and North America, while genotype 1b is predominantly found in Southern and Eastern Europe and Japan. Genotype 2 is less common than genotype 1 and is found more in Europe than in North America. Genotype 3 is endemic in Southeast Asia, and genotype 4 is characteristic for the Middle East, Egypt, and central Africa. Genotype 5 is almost exclusively found in South Africa, and genotypes 6 to 11 are mostly

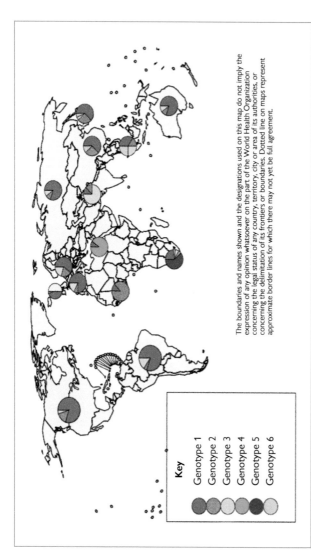

Figure 2.2 Geographic distribution of hepatitis C genotype worldwide, 2009. (Data from World Health Organization. Available at: http://www.who.int/vaccine_research/documents/ViralCancer7.pdf. Accessed July 16, 2011.)

The boundaries and names shown and the designations used on this map do not imply the expression of any opinion whatsoever on the part of the World Health Organization concerning the legal status of any country, territory, city or area of its authorities, or concerning the delimitation of its frontiers or boundaries. Dotted line on maps represent approximate border lines for which there may not yet be full agreement.

Key
Genotype 1
Genotype 2
Genotype 3
Genotype 4
Genotype 5
Genotype 6

distributed in Asia (Global surveillance, 1999; Houghton, 1996; Mondelli & Silini, 1999; Nguyen & Keeffe, 2005; Recommendations, 1998).

The impact of viral genotype in the pathogenesis of liver disease remains a subject of controversy, but the influence of the genotype in the response to interferon-based therapy is established. Genotype 1 is generally associated with a poorer response to therapy, while genotypes 2 and 3 have a more favorable response. Genotype 4 appears to have an intermediate response (Kamal & Nasser, 2008; Nguyen & Keeffe, 2005).

In the United States, genotype 1 predominates in 79% of the viremic individuals (58% for genotype 1a and 21% for genotype 1b). Genotype 2 were detected in 15% (2% for genotype 2a and 13% for genotype 2b), genotype 3 in 5%, and genotype 4a in 1% (Zein et al., 1996). A similar distribution was reported in a larger study of 6,807 patients, with genotype 1 detected in 73% , genotype 2 in 14%, genotype 3 in 8%, mixed genotype in 4%, and genotypes 4, 5, and 6 in <1% (Blatt et al., 2000).

Epidemiology in the United States

The prevalence of HCV infection in the United States has been estimated from the National Health and Nutrition Examination Survey (NHANES). NHANES III data gathered from 1988 to 1994 estimated that 1.8% of the U.S. population, or 3.9 million individuals, were exposed to hepatitis C as detected by serum HCV antibody, and that 70% of exposed persons, or 2.7 million individuals, harbored the virus chronically (Alter, 1999). An analysis of more recent NHANES data from 1999 to 2002 by Armstrong and colleagues (2006) reported a similar overall prevalence of HCV exposure at 1.6%, or 4.1 million individuals, and an estimated prevalence of chronic infection at 1.3%, or 3.2 million individuals. The infection is more common in men (2.1%) than women (1.1%), and in non-Hispanic Blacks (3%) than in non-Hispanic Whites (1.5%) and Mexican Americans (1.3%). It is present in 1.0% of individuals age 20 to 29 years, peaks in prevalence at 4.3% in the 40-to-49-year age group, and decreases to 1.6% in individuals 50 to 59 years of age and to 0.9% in persons 60 years or older. These findings represent an upward shift of the peak age group from the 35-to-39 age group in the previous NHANES III study, as expected with aging of this group. Most individuals with HCV infection were born between 1945 and 1964 (Armstrong et al., 2006).

The survey, however, failed to assess the homeless or incarcerated, so the true prevalence of HCV infection in the United States is probably higher. HCV antibodies were detected in 41.7% of homeless veterans were tested for HCV antibody, with intravenous drug use identified as a major risk factor (Cheung et al., 2002). In 2004, there were 2.4 million individuals incarcerated in the United States. These individuals similarly have a high prevalence of HCV exposure, with estimates at 12% to 35% of prisoners (Weinbaum et al., 2005). Two recent meta-analyses place the prevalence at about 30% to 40% of inmates (Gough et al., 2010; Vescio et al., 2008). About 30% of HCV-infected individuals spend time in a correctional facility, and intravenous drug use is named as the most common risk factor. Interestingly, women inmates had higher prevalence rates than men, contrary to the general HCV-infected population, and this may be due to the higher rate at which women are incarcerated for behaviors associated with increased risk for HCV, such as intravenous drug use and prostitution (Vescio et al., 2008).

Prior to the implementation of universal screening of blood donors in 1992, the predominant mode of transmission in the general HCV-infected population was exposure to infected blood and blood products. The enhanced screening of blood products has led to a decline of the estimated incidence of acute hepatitis C from 180,000 in the mid-1980s to an estimated 16,000 in 2009 (CDC, Disease burden). Currently, intravenous drug use and high-risk sexual exposures account for most HCV transmission (Alter, 2007; Armstrong et al., 2006).

While new cases of HCV infection have declined substantially over the past 25 years, from 7.4 per 100,000 individuals during 1982 to 1989 to 0.7 per 100,000 individuals during 1994 to 2006 (Williams et al., 2011), the prevalence of chronic infections for more than 20 years is expected to increase (Alter, 2007). Despite this, HCV infection remains underdiagnosed in populations who are at risk (Table 2.1). The main impediment to the prevention and control of HCV is lack of knowledge and awareness about this disease among healthcare and social-service providers, the lay community, and policymakers (CDC, Hepatitis C information; Mitchell et al., 2010). Awareness and access to the diagnosis and treatment of HCV infection need to be addressed adequately.

Table 2.1 Who Should Be Tested for HCV Infection?
Persons who have ever injected illegal drugs, including those who have injected only once many years ago
Recipients of clotting factor concentrates made before 1987
Recipients of blood products or solid organ transplants before 1992
Patients who have ever received long-term hemodialysis therapy
Persons such as healthcare workers with known exposures to HCV, such as needlesticks
Recipients of blood products or organs from a donor who later tested positive for HCV
All HIV-infected persons
Children born to HCV-infected mothers (HCV antibody should be tested after 18 months to avoid detecting maternal antibody)
Adapted from CDC. *Hepatitis C information for health professionals.* Available at: http://www.cdc.gov/hepatitis/HCV/HCVfaq.htm (Accessed on July 16, 2011).

References

Alter, M. J. (2007). Epidemiology of hepatitis C virus infection. *World Journal of Gastroenterology, 13,* 2436–2441.

Alter, M. J., D. Kruzon-Moran, O. V. Nainan, G. M. McQuillan, F. Gao, L. A. Moyer, et al. (1999). The Prevalence of Hepatitis C Virus Infection in the United States, 1988 through 1994. *The New England Journal of Medicine,* 341, 556–562.

Armstrong, G. L., A. Wasley, E. P. Simard, G. M. McQuillan, W. L. Kuhnert, & M. J. Alter (2006). The prevalence of hepatitis C virus infection in the United States, 1999 through 2002. *Annals of Internal Medicine, 144,* 705–714.

Blatt, L. M., M. G. Mutchnick, M. J. Tong, F. M. Klion, E. Lebovics, B. Freilich, et al. (2000). Assessment of hepatitis C virus RNA and genotype from 6807 patients with chronic hepatitis C in the United States. *Journal of Viral Hepatitis,* 7, 196–202.

CDC. *Disease Burden from Hepatitis A, B and C.* Available at: http://www.cdc.gov/ hepatitis/PDFs/disease_burden.pdf. Accessed on April 29, 2012

CDC. *Hepatitis C Information for Health Professionals.* Available at: http://www.cdc. gov/hepatitis/HCV/HCVfaq.htm. Accessed on July 16, 2011.

Cheung, R. C., A. K. Hanson, K. Maganti, E. B. Keeffe, & S. M. Matsui (2002). Viral hepatitis and other infectious diseases in a homeless population. *Journal of Clinical Gastroenterology, 34,* 476–480.

EASL International Consensus Conference on Hepatitis C. (1999). Consensus Statement. *Journal of Hepatology, 31,* 3–8.

(1999). Global surveillance and control of hepatitis C. Report of a WHO Consultation organized in collaboration with the Viral Hepatitis Prevention Board, Antwerp, Belgium. *Journal of Viral Hepatitis,* 6, 35–47.

Gough, E., M. C. Kempf, L. Graham, M. Manzanero, E. W. Hook, A. Bartolucci, et al. (2010). HIV and hepatitis B and C incidence rates in US correctional populations and high risk groups: a systematic review and meta-analysis. *BMC Public Health, 10,* 777.

Houghton, M. (1996). Hepatitis C viruses. In: B. N. Fields, D. M. Knipe, & P. M. (Eds.), *Fields Virology* (3rd ed., pp. 1036–1058). Philadelphia: Lippincott-Raven.

Kamal, S. M., & I. A. Nasser (2008). Hepatitis C genotype 4: What we know and what we don't yet know. *Hepatology, 47,* 1371–1383.

Mitchell, A. E., H. M. Colvin, & R. Palmer Beasley. (2010). Institute of Medicine recommendations for the prevention and control of hepatitis B and C. *Hepatology, 51,* 729–733.

Mondelli, M. U., & E. Silini (1999). Clinical significance of hepatitis C virus genotypes. *Journal of Hepatology, 31*(Suppl 1), 65–70.

Nguyen, M. H., & E. B. Keeffe (2005). Chronic hepatitis C: genotypes 4 to 9. *Clinics in Liver Disease, 9,* 411–426.

Perz, J. F., G. L. Armstrong, L. A. Farrington, Y. J. Hutin, & B. P. Bell (2006). The contributions of hepatitis B virus and hepatitis C virus infections to cirrhosis and primary liver cancer worldwide. *Journal of Hepatology, 45,* 529–538.

(1998). Recommendations for prevention and control of hepatitis C virus (HCV) infection and HCV related chronic disease. *MMWR,* 47.

van der Poel, C. L. (1999). Hepatitis C virus and blood transfusion: past and present risks. *Journal of Hepatology, 31*(Suppl 1), 101–106.

Vescio, M. F., B. Longo, S. Babudieri, G. Starnini, S. Carbonara, G. Rezza, et al. (2008). Correlates of hepatitis C virus seropositivity in prison inmates: a meta-analysis. *Journal of Epidemiology and Community Health, 62,* 305–313.

Weinbaum, C. M., K. M. Sabin, & S. S. Santibanez (2005). Hepatitis B, hepatitis C, and HIV in correctional populations: a review of epidemiology and prevention. *AIDS, 19*(Suppl 3), S41–46.

WHO. *Hepatitis C.* WHO Fact Sheet No. 164, Revised 2000. Available at: http://www.who.int/mediacentre/factsheets/fs164/en/. Accessed on March 8, 2009.

Williams, I. T., B. P. Bell, W. Kuhnert, & M. J. Alter. (2011). Incidence and transmission patterns of acute hepatitis C in the United States, 1982–2006. *Archives of Internal Medicine, 171,* 242–248.

Zein, N. N., J. Rakela, E. L. Krawitt, K. R. Reddy, T. Tominaga, & D. H. Persing. (1996). Hepatitis C virus genotypes in the United States: epidemiology, pathogenicity, and response to interferon therapy. Collaborative Study Group. *Annals of Internal Medicine, 125,* 634–639.

Chapter 3

Natural History of Hepatitis C

Erin Jenkins and Andrew Aronsohn

Introduction

Hepatitis C virus (HCV) is the most common cause of death from liver disease in the United States (Ghany et al., 2009). This chapter reviews the natural history of hepatitis C, from transmission to the development of chronic liver disease and its associated complications.

Risk Factors for Transmission

Hepatitis C is transmitted through intravenous drug use (IVDU), blood and blood product transfusions, and less commonly through sexual intercourse, vertical transmission by HCV-infected mothers, and healthcare-related exposures (Fig. 3.1). Individuals with repeated direct percutaneous exposures or those with large-volume exposures have a higher prevalence of HCV, while those with infrequent small-volume exposures or mucosal contact have much lower prevalence rates (Fig. 3.2).

Illicit Drug and Other Behavioral Transmission

IVDU still accounts for approximately half of all cases of acute hepatitis C in the United States; however, rates of IVDU and incidence of hepatitis C virus have decreased over recent years (Williams et al., 2011) (Fig. 3.3). The prevalence of HCV among patients who use IV drugs ranges from 35% to 80% (Amon et al., 2008; CDC, 1998). Risk of HCV is highest among those who have greater than 5 years of IVDU, those with daily IVDU, and those who inject both heroin and cocaine (Amon et al., 2008). HCV can also be transmitted through intranasal cocaine use and shared paraphernalia. When proper hygienic techniques are not employed, HCV can be transmitted through cosmetic procedures such as piercings and tattoos, as well as through complementary treatments such as acupuncture.

Sexual Transmission

Although sexual transmission of HCV does occur, the virus is transmitted inefficiently through sexual contact, and the rate of transmission among long-term sexual partners is low. The seroconversion rate among monogamous heterosexual partners where one person is infected is less than 1% annually (Tahan

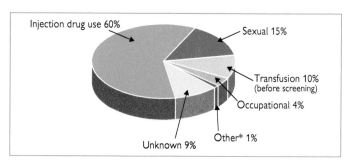

Figure 3.1 Sources of infection for persons with viral hepatitis C (http://www.chronicliverdisease.org/library/slide/slide_topic.cfm?topic=ed3_epidemiology, Slide 13)

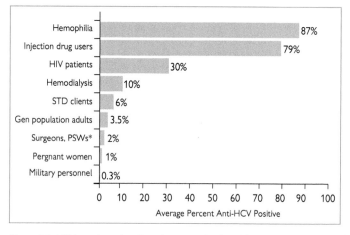

Figure 3.2 HCV prevalence by selected groups in the United States (http://www.chronicliverdisease.org/library/slide/slide_topic.cfm?topic=ed3_epidemiology, Slide 14)

et al., 2005). The prevalence of hepatitis C among spouses of HCV-positive persons is 1.5% to 5%, though shared high-risk behaviors may also contribute to this number (CDC, 1998; Thomas et al., 1995). Due to the low rate of transmission among monogamous partners, the CDC does not specifically recommend initiating barrier protection among monogamous partners. Household members should avoid sharing razors, toothbrushes, or other items that could lead to percutaneous exposure to blood (CDC, 1998).

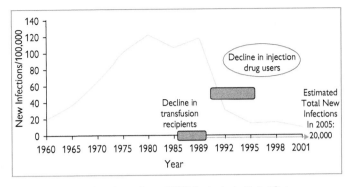

Figure 3.3 Estimated incidence of acute HCV infection in the United States, 1960–2001 (http://www.chronicliverdisease.org/library/slide/slide_topic.cfm?topic= ed3_epidemiology, Slide 8)

Persons with high-risk sexual behaviors such as unprotected sex and multiple lifetime sexual partners have higher rates of hepatitis C. As is the case with other sexually transmitted infections, females may be at higher risk for contracting the infection sexually. HIV-infected men who have sex with men, especially those who engage in sexual behaviors that increase mucosal trauma, are also at increased risk for infection with hepatitis C (Sexual transmission, 2011; Taylor et al., 2011).

Vertical Transmission

Maternal–fetal transmission, also known as vertical transmission, is rare and occurs almost exclusively in women with detectable viral load. The fetal transmission rate is estimated at 5% in infants born to women with positive HCV RNA, but the transmission rate is increased to19.4% among infants born to women who are co-infected with HIV (Indolfi & Resti, 2009). The timing and mode of transmission from mother to child remain unclear. Data from one prospective cohort study suggest that at least one third of infected infants acquired infection *in utero*, with intrapartum and peripartum infection accounting for other infections (Mok et al., 2005). Prolonged rupture of membranes, vaginal lacerations, and procedures that expose the fetus to maternal blood, such as fetal scalp monitors, all may increase the risk of transmission.

Few measures can be taken to reduce the risk of vertical transmission of HCV, especially since treatment of HCV is contraindicated during pregnancy. Delivery by elective cesarean section has not been shown to reduce the rate of infection (Ghamar Chehreh et al., 2011). HCV is not transmitted through breast milk, despite low levels of HCV present in milk, and therefore infected women may breastfeed in the absence of skin or nipple breakdown that would expose the infant to blood (Indolfi & Resti, 2009). All infants born to HCV-antibody-positive mothers should be tested for HCV, though testing should be deferred until 18 months to avoid the detection of passively transferred maternal anti-HCV (CDC, 1998).

Nosocomial Transmission

While blood transfusion was identified as a likely source of infection in 15% of acute hepatitis C cases in 1982, subsequent improvements in donor and blood screening techniques have reduced the risk greatly. In the 1960s, 20% of patients receiving transfusion experienced a post-transfusion hepatitis, of which the vast majority of cases were non-A, non-B hepatitis, later identified as hepatitis C. Changes in donor screening were initiated in 1978, including the transition to a volunteer-only donor pool and the addition of donor exclusion criteria, decreasing the risk of post-transfusion hepatitis. Universal testing for anti-HCV was initiated in 1990, and blood transfusions have accounted for less than 2% of HCV infections after 1992. The addition of nucleic acid testing for HCV in 1999 further decreased the risk of acquiring hepatitis C from blood transfusion, which is currently estimated at only 1 in 2 million units transfused. Persons with hemophilia who received concentrated clotting factors prior to 1989 had a greater than 90% prevalence of HCV (CDC, 1998). Beginning in 1989, viral inactivation procedures were initiated, dramatically decreasing the risk of viral exposure. Still, the prevalence of HCV in this population remains high due to the chronicity of disease.

Healthcare-related epidemics of hepatitis C are rare but have been reported in both hospital and outpatient settings due to failure to comply with recommended sterilization techniques, including improper reuse of syringes and multiuse medication vials in addition to improperly cleaned environmental surfaces at dialysis centers (Thompson et al., 2009). The risk of HCV transmission to a healthcare provider is as high as 10% with a needlestick injury from an infected patient, and may be further increased when the patient's viral load exceeds 500,000 (Sulkowski et al., 2002).

Host Response to HCV

Acute Hepatitis C

Only 15% to 30% of people who acquire hepatitis C virus will develop clinically recognizable acute hepatitis C, manifested by acute onset of malaise, jaundice, influenza-like symptoms, elevated aminotransferase levels, and serologic evidence of hepatitis C infection (Williams et al., 2011). Symptom onset may be days to weeks after exposure. Fulminant hepatitis C is exceedingly rare, and mortality among those with acute hepatitis C is less than 1% (Williams et al., 2011) (Fig. 3.4).

Testing and Serologies

Hepatitis C RNA is detectable by assays as early as 2 weeks after exposure to the virus, while anti-HCV does not become detectable until approximately

HCA RNA first detected in blood	1–3 weeks
Time until symptoms (if any)	Average 6–7 weeks Range 2–26 weeks
Antibody first detected in blood	In 50–70% at onset of symptoms; in 90% by 3 months
Acute illness (jaundice) Chronic infection (mostly asx) Cirrhosis	Mild (≤ 20%) 75%–85% 10%–20%
Mortality from CLD	1%–5%

Figure 3.4 Features of hepatitis C virus infection (http://www.chronicliverdisease.org/library/slide/slide_topic.cfm?topic=ed3_epidemiology, Slide 35)

8 to 12 weeks after exposure (Hofer et al., 2003). Thus, screening using anti-HCV only may not detect those who have acquired HCV infection within the previous 8 to 12 weeks, also known as a "window period." Individuals who clear hepatitis C virus will have undetectable HCV RNA but will remain anti-HCV positive. Individuals with positive HCV RNA and anti- HCV in the absence of an acute infection or with anti-HCV and HCV RNA persistent more than 6 months after the acute infection meet the criteria for chronic hepatitis C (Figs. 3.5a and 3.5b).

Factors Affecting Spontaneous Clearance of the Virus

The majority of patients with acute hepatitis C infection will develop chronic hepatitis C (CHC), though certain populations have higher rates of spontaneous clearance of the virus. Specifically, women and children appear to have higher rates of clearance. An Irish study investigating young women with hepatitis C exposures from contaminated anti-D immunoglobulin demonstrated a clearance rate of 45% (Kenny-Walsh, 1999). Similarly, 45% of children infected with hepatitis C after perioperative blood transfusions spontaneously cleared the virus (Vogt et al., 1999). Jaundice, though present in less than 10% of infections, is a clinical marker for a robust host immune response, and is associated with a higher rate of spontaneous clearance of the virus (Hofer et al., 2003; Maheshwari et al., 2008). Increased spontaneous clearance also occurs more frequently in individuals infected with HCV genotype 3. Genome-wide association studies have identified rs12979860 polymorphism, located 3 kb upstream from the IL28b gene, as an important predictor of response to standard interferon therapy. Those with the favorable C/C genotype are three times more likely to spontaneously clear the virus than those with the T/T polymorphism (Thomas et al., 2009). IL 28b has also been shown to be an important predictor of viral clearance among infants with perinatal exposures to hepatitis C (Ruiz-Extremera et al., 2011).

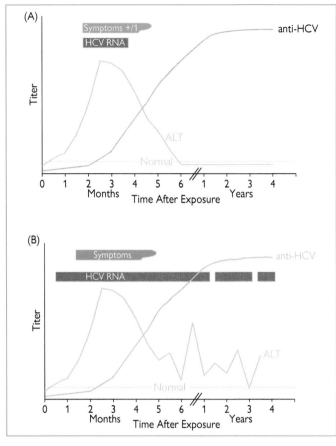

Figure 3.5 Serologic pattern of acute HCV infection if recovery (A) and with progression to chronic infection (B) (http://www.chronicliverdisease.org/library/slide/slide_topic.cfm?topic=ed3_epidemiology, Slides 36 [A] and 37 [B])

Chronic Hepatitis C

Overall, 65% to 80% of people infected with hepatitis C will develop chronic disease (Armstrong et al., 2006). Patients with CHC are often asymptomatic prior to developing cirrhosis, or may exhibit symptoms such as fatigue, myalgias or arthralgias, weight loss, anorexia, and mental slowing. Extrahepatic manifestations of hepatitis C such as cryoglobulinemia and porphyria cutanea tarda are secondary to effects of the virus, and can occur in the absence of liver disease. The rate of progression to cirrhosis varies from individual to individual, but in general occurs over decades. Approximately 16% of patients develop cirrhosis at 20 years postinfection, with 41% developing cirrhosis by 30 years (Thein et al., 2008). Hepatic decompensation, including variceal bleeding, ascites, encephalopathy, and jaundice, occurs in one third of patients with HCV cirrhosis for over 10 years (Planas et al., 2004). Five-year survival in those who have experienced some manifestation of hepatic decompensation is approximately 50% (Planas et al., 2004) (Fig. 3.6).

Factors Affecting Disease Progression

Only 20% to 40% of those with CHC progress to cirrhosis. The variability in liver-related morbidity and mortality caused by HCV can be at least partially explained by host and viral factors that play a role in progression of hepatitis C to advanced liver disease (Table 3.1).

Fibrosis to Cirrhosis

Chronic HCV infection causes inflammation and injury, resulting in fibrogenesis. Fibrosis is characterized by deposition of collagen and extracellular matrix proteins, resulting in loss of liver architecture and ultimately cirrhosis. Biopsy is the gold standard for evaluating fibrosis, although serum markers are also used to estimate the degree of fibrosis. Cross-sectional studies have shown that fibrosis progresses in a relatively linear fashion, with median time to cirrhosis of 30 years. However, rates of progression to fibrosis are not normally distributed, with patients separating into groups of slow, intermediate, and rapid progressors (Poynard et al., 1997) (Fig. 3.7). Host and viral factors play a role in the rate of progression of disease and are discussed below.

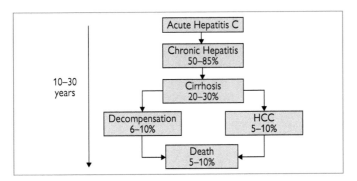

Figure 3.6 Natural history of hepatitis C (http://www.chronicliverdisease.org/library/slide/slide_topic.cfm?topic=ed3_epidemiology, Slide 39)

Table 3.1 Factors Associated with Accelerated Disease Progression

- HIV co-infection
- Hepatitis B co-infection
- Infection with HCV genotype 3
- Older age at time of infection (age >50)
- Male gender
- Chronic alcohol consumption
- Chronic marijuana use
- Obesity and insulin resistance
- Genetic factors (under investigation)

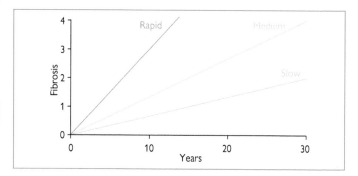

Figure 3.7 Modeling of liver fibrosis in HCV: different rates of progression (http://www.chronicliverdisease.org/library/slide/slide_topic.cfm?topic=ed3_epidemiology, Slide 45)

Demographic factors

Age

Children and young women have been shown to have lower rates of progression to cirrhosis as well as increased rates of spontaneous viral clearance (Kenny-Walsh, 1999; Vogt et al., 1999). Alternatively, acquiring the disease at an older age (after age 40 to 50) is associated with an accelerated progression of liver injury (Poynard et al., 1997; Seeff, 1997). Cross-sectional studies have shown age to be an independent predictor of fibrosis progression, and progression is most rapid in those infected after age 50 (Poynard et al., 1997, 2001). Even among those infected at a younger age, cirrhosis progression is still accelerated after reaching age 50 (Poynard et al., 2001). The mechanisms behind the increased progression are still not fully elucidated. The aging liver is less able to adapt to injury, and age-related changes in hepatocyte proliferation and response to oxidative stress have been noted (Hoare et al., 2010). Further, aged persons demonstrate a significant decline in immune response, particularly in relation to T cells, and this host–virus interaction may also play a role (Solana & Pawelec, 1998). The peak incidence of hepatitis C occurred between 1970 and 1990, and as that population ages and suffers disease progression, the prevalence of HCV cirrhosis is expected to increase and peak in 2020 (Davis et al., 2010).

Race

African Americans, despite having a higher liver-related mortality than whites, appear to have a slower rate of progression of fibrosis (Crosse et al., 2004; Sterling et al., 2004; Wiley et al., 2002). Data comparing progression among other races is not as robust, though it appears to be accelerated in non-black American Hispanics as compared to whites (Missiha et al., 2008).

Behavioral Factors

Alcohol consumption in the setting of chronic HCV has been associated with a twofold increased risk of progression to cirrhosis and HCC and of overall mortality. Its use, even at moderate levels, is associated with increased HCV RNA levels and higher rates of fibrosis (Kyrlagkitsis et al., 2002; Martinot-Peignoux et al., 2001; Puoti et al., 2002). A safe amount of alcohol use has not been established for those with CHC; therefore, abstinence from alcohol is recommended. Chronic daily marijuana use and tobacco smoking have also been shown to increase the rate of progression of steatosis and fibrosis (Hezode et al., 2005).

Metabolic Factors

Metabolic factors, including obesity and insulin resistance, likely adversely effect outcomes in CHC. This was demonstrated in patients with insulin resistance and evidence of baseline steatosis, who were shown to be at increased risk of histologic progression of fibrosis and complications of cirrhosis (Everhart et al., 2009). Small studies have shown improvement in aminotransferase levels with weight loss among obese patients with chronic liver disease, suggesting that a weight-loss program would be a reasonable intervention (Hickman et al., 2004).

Co-infections

Patients who are co-infected with HIV have higher HCV RNA levels and more rapid progression to cirrhosis. Up to one fourth of patients with HIV are co-infected with hepatitis C, due to overlapping risk factors and an impaired immune response that decreases clearance rates. A low CD4 count portends a fourfold relative risk of hepatic decompensation (Pineda et al., 2007). To date, there is no evidence that early initiation of highly active antiretroviral therapy (HAART) in co-infected patients delays progression (Pineda et al., 2007). Co-infection with HBV or with multiple strains of HCV also results in increased disease progression. Thus, abstaining from high-risk behaviors such as IVDU, even after acquiring chronic hepatitis C, is prudent (Missiha et al., 2008). Patients should be screened for HIV and hepatitis B at the time of diagnosis to allow for immunization of those who are not immune to HBV and consideration for HIV treatment.

Viral Factors

Although HCV genotype plays a crucial role in treatment outcomes, only genotype 3 is independently associated with increased progression of liver disease. However, it is also linked with increased steatosis, and it is hypothesized that the increased steatosis is the predominant reason for accelerated disease progression (Missiha et al., 2008).

Genetic Factors

IL28b, though important in spontaneous clearance of the virus, has not been shown to affect disease progression (Marabita et al., 2011). Various other target gene polymorphisms have been investigated, including HLA classes, profibrogenic cytokines, and PNPLA3 (Trepo et al., 2011). One genome-wide association study identified seven SNPS that in combination were predictors of cirrhosis, though further investigation in the role of host genetics in disease progression is needed (Huang et al., 2007).

Hepatocellular Carcinoma

Hepatitis C-related cirrhosis accounts for approximately one third of HCC cases in the United States. Almost all hepatitis C-related HCC is found in the setting of cirrhosis, in which the incidence is estimated to be between 2% and 8% per year (Degos et al., 2000; Fattovich et al., 1997). As medical care for end-stage liver disease improves and affected individuals live longer, HCC has become an important indication for liver transplantation. Alcohol use, obesity, and insulin resistance have also been linked to HCC and may affect the development of HCC among individuals with HCV.

CHC and Survival

Chronic HCV infection is associated with a 2.37-times higher mortality rate ratio than healthy controls and a 26-fold increase in liver-related mortality (El-Kamary et al., 2011). Interestingly, those with positive anti-HCV without CHC still had a 1.79-times higher mortality rate. Behavioral and lifestyle risks that predispose to HCV exposure may also contribute to non-liver-related mortality increase. Among a group of individuals with compensated cirrhosis, 5- and 10-year transplant-free survival rates were 91% and 79%, respectively (Fattovich et al., 1997). Five-year survival after liver transplantation for CHC is approximately 70% (Ghobrial et al., 2001).

Conclusion

Chronic hepatitis C is a common cause of liver disease worldwide. As therapeutic interventions for CHC continue to improve, continued focus on the natural history of the disease will be a key component in reducing overall liver-related morbidity and mortality.

References

Amon, J. J., R. S. Garfein, L. Ahdieh-Grant, et al. (2008). Prevalence of hepatitis C virus infection among injection drug users in the United States, 1994–2004. *Clinical Infectious Diseases, 46*(12), 1852–1858.

Armstrong, G. L., A. Wasley, E. P. Simard, G. M. McQuillan, W. L. Kuhnert, & M. J. Alter (2006). The prevalence of hepatitis C virus infection in the United States, 1999 through 2002. *Annals of Internal Medicine, 144*(10), 705–714.

CDC (1998). Recommendations for prevention and control of hepatitis C virus (HCV) infection and HCV-related chronic disease. *MMWR Recomm Rep, 47* (RR-19), 1–39.

Crosse, K., O. G. Umeadi, F. A. Anania, et al. (2004). Racial differences in liver inflammation and fibrosis related to chronic hepatitis C. *Clinical Gastroenterology and Hepatology, 2*(6), 463–468.

Davis, G. L., M. J. Alter, H. El-Serag, T. Poynard, & L. W. Jennings. (2010). Aging of hepatitis C virus (HCV)-infected persons in the United States: a multiple cohort model of HCV prevalence and disease progression. *Gastroenterology, 138*(2), 513–521.

Degos, F., C. Christidis, N. Ganne-Carrie, et al. (2000). Hepatitis C virus-related cirrhosis: time to occurrence of hepatocellular carcinoma and death. *Gut, 47*(1), 131–136.

El-Kamary, S. S., R. Jhaveri, & M. D. Shardell. (2011). All-cause, liver-related, and non-liver-related mortality among HCV-infected individuals in the general US population. *Clinical Infectious Diseases, 53*(2), 150–157.

Everhart, J. E., A. S. Lok, H. Y. Kim, et al. (2009). Weight-related effects on disease progression in the hepatitis C antiviral long-term treatment against cirrhosis trial. *Gastroenterology, 137*(2), 549–557.

Fattovich, G., G. Giustina, F. Degos, et al. (1997). Morbidity and mortality in compensated cirrhosis type C: a retrospective follow-up study of 384 patients. *Gastroenterology, 112*(2), 463–472.

Ghamar Chehreh, M. E., S. V. Tabatabaei, S. Khazanehdari, & S. M. Alavian. (2011). Effect of cesarean section on the risk of perinatal transmission of hepatitis C virus from HCV-RNA+/HIV- mothers: a meta-analysis. *Archives of Gynecology Obstetrics, 283*(2), 255–260.

Ghany, M. G., D. B. Strader, D. L. Thomas, & L. B. Seeff. (2009). Diagnosis, management, and treatment of hepatitis C: an update. *Hepatology, 49*(4), 1335–1374.

Ghobrial, R. M., R. Steadman, J. Gornbein, et al. (2001). A 10-year experience of liver transplantation for hepatitis C: analysis of factors determining outcome in over 500 patients. *Annals of Surgery, 234*(3), 384–393.

Hezode, C., F. Roudot-Thoraval, S. Nguyen, et al. (2005). Daily cannabis smoking as a risk factor for progression of fibrosis in chronic hepatitis C. *Hepatology, 42*(1), 63–71.

Hickman, I. J., J. R. Jonsson, J. B. Prins, et al. (2004). Modest weight loss and physical activity in overweight patients with chronic liver disease results in sustained improvements in alanine aminotransferase, fasting insulin, and quality of life. *Gut, 53*(3), 413–419.

Hoare, M., T. Das, & G. Alexander. (2010). Ageing, telomeres, senescence, and liver injury. *Journal of Hepatology, 53*(5), 950–961.

Hofer, H., T. Watkins-Riedel, O. Janata, et al. (2003). Spontaneous viral clearance in patients with acute hepatitis C can be predicted by repeated measurements of serum viral load. *Hepatology, 37*(1), 60–64.

Huang, H., M. L. Shiffman, S. Friedman, et al. (2007). A 7 gene signature identifies the risk of developing cirrhosis in patients with chronic hepatitis C. *Hepatology, 46*(2), 297–306.

Indolfi, G., & M. Resti (2009). Perinatal transmission of hepatitis C virus infection. *Journal of Medical Virology, 81*(5), 836–843.

Kenny-Walsh, E. (1999). Clinical outcomes after hepatitis C infection from contaminated anti-D immune globulin. Irish Hepatology Research Group. *New England Journal of Medicine, 340*(16), 1228–1233.

Kyrlagkitsis, I., B. Portmann, H. Smith, J. O'Grady, & M. E. Cramp (2003). Liver histology and progression of fibrosis in individuals with chronic hepatitis C and persistently normal ALT. *American Journal of Gastroenterology, 98*(7), 1588–1593.

Maheshwari, A., S. Ray, & P. J. Thuluvath. (2008). Acute hepatitis C. *Lancet, 372*(9635), 321–332.

Marabita, F., A. Aghemo, S. De Nicola, et al. (June 30, 2011). Genetic variation in IL28B gene is not associated with fibrosis progression in patients with chronic hepatitis C and known date of infection. *Hepatology.* doi: 10.1002/hep.24503.

Martinot-Peignoux, M., N. Boyer, D. Cazals-Hatem, et al. (2001). Prospective study on anti-hepatitis C virus-positive patients with persistently normal serum alanine transaminase with or without detectable serum hepatitis C virus RNA. *Hepatology, 34*(5), 1000–1005.

Missiha, S. B., M. Ostrowski, & E. J. Heathcote. (2008). Disease progression in chronic hepatitis C: modifiable and nonmodifiable factors. *Gastroenterology, 134*(6), 1699–1714.

Mok, J., L. Pembrey, P. A. Tovo, & M. L. Newell (2005). When does mother to child transmission of hepatitis C virus occur? *Archives of Disease in Childhood Fetal Neonatal Edition, 90*(2), F156–160.

Pineda, J. A., J. A. Garcia-Garcia, M. Aguilar-Guisado, et al. (2007). Clinical progression of hepatitis C virus-related chronic liver disease in human immunodeficiency virus-infected patients undergoing highly active antiretroviral therapy. *Hepatology, 46*(3), 622–630.

Planas, R., B. Balleste, M. A. Alvarez, et al. (2004). Natural history of decompensated hepatitis C virus-related cirrhosis. A study of 200 patients. *Journal of Hepatology, 40*(5), 823–830.

Puoti, C., R. Castellacci, F. Montagnese, et al. (2002). Histological and virological features and follow-up of hepatitis C virus carriers with normal aminotransferase levels: the Italian prospective study of the asymptomatic C carriers (ISACC). *Journal of Hepatology, 37*(1), 117–123.

Poynard, T., P. Bedossa, & P. Opolon P. (1997). Natural history of liver fibrosis progression in patients with chronic hepatitis C. The OBSVIRC, METAVIR, CLINIVIR, and DOSVIRC groups. *Lancet, 349*(9055), 825–832.

Poynard, T., V. Ratziu, F. Charlotte, Z. Goodman, J. McHutchison, & J. Albrecht. (2001). Rates and risk factors of liver fibrosis progression in patients with chronic hepatitis C. *Journal of Hepatology, 34*(5), 730–739.

Ruiz-Extremera, A., J. A. Munoz-Gamez, M. A. Salmeron-Ruiz, et al. (2011). Genetic variation in interleukin 28B with respect to vertical transmission of hepatitis C virus and spontaneous clearance in HCV-infected children. *Hepatology, 53*(6), 1830–1838.

Seeff, L. B. (1997). Natural history of hepatitis C. *Hepatology, 26*(3 Suppl 1), 21S–28S.

(July 22, 2011). Sexual transmission of hepatitis C virus among HIV-infected men who have sex with men—New York City, 2005–2010. *MMWR Morbidity Mortality Weekly Report, 60,* 945–950.

Solana, R., & G. Pawelec. (1998). Molecular and cellular basis of immunosenescence. *Mechanisms of Ageing and Development, 102*(2-3), 115–129.

Sterling, R. K., R. T. Stravitz, V. A. Luketic, et al. (2004). A comparison of the spectrum of chronic hepatitis C virus between Caucasians and African Americans. *Clinical Gastroenterology and Hepatology, 2*(6), 469–473.

Sulkowski, M. S., S. C. Ray, & D. L. Thomas. (2002). Needlestick transmission of hepatitis C. *Journal of the American Medical Association, 287*(18), 2406–2413.

Tahan, V., C. Karaca, B. Yildirim, et al. (2005). Sexual transmission of HCV between spouses. *American Journal of Gastroenterology, 100*(4), 821–824.

Taylor, L. E., M. Holubar, K. Wu, et al. (2011). Incident hepatitis C virus infection among US HIV-infected men enrolled in clinical trials. *Clinical Infectious Diseases, 52*(6), 812–818.

Thein, H. H., Q. Yi, G. J. Dore, & M. D. Krahn. (2008). Estimation of stage-specific fibrosis progression rates in chronic hepatitis C virus infection: a meta-analysis and meta-regression. *Hepatology, 48*(2), 418–431.

Thomas, D. L., C. L. Thio, M. P. Martin, et al. (2009). Genetic variation in IL28B and spontaneous clearance of hepatitis C virus. *Nature, 461*(7265), 798–801.

Thomas, D. L., J. M. Zenilman, H. J. Alter, et al. (1995). Sexual transmission of hepatitis C virus among patients attending sexually transmitted diseases clinics in Baltimore—an analysis of 309 sex partnerships. *Journal of Infectious Disease, 171*(4), 768–775.

Thompson, N. D., J. F. Perz, A. C. Moorman, & S. D. Holmberg. (2009). Nonhospital health care-associated hepatitis B and C virus transmission: United States, 1998–2008. *Annals of Internal Medicine, 150*(1), 33–39.

Trepo, E., P. Pradat, A. Potthoff, et al. (2011). Impact of patatin-like phospholipase-3 (rs738409 C>G) polymorphism on fibrosis progression and steatosis in chronic hepatitis C. *Hepatology, 54*(1), 60–69.

Vogt, M., T. Lang, G. Frosner, et al. (1999). Prevalence and clinical outcome of hepatitis C infection in children who underwent cardiac surgery before the implementation of blood-donor screening. *New England Journal of Medicine, 341*(12), 866–870.

Wiley, T. E., J. Brown, & J. Chan. (2002). Hepatitis C infection in African Americans: its natural history and histological progression. *American Journal of Gastroenterology, 97*(3), 700–706.

Williams, I. T., B. P. Bell, W. Kuhnert, & M. J. Alter. (2011). Incidence and transmission patterns of acute hepatitis C in the United States, 1982–2006. *Archives of Internal Medicine, 171*(3), 242–248.

Chapter 4

Diagnostic Testing

Natasha Walzer and Scott Cotler

The initial evaluation for hepatitis C virus infection (HCV) encompasses both the decision to screen an individual for the disease and the evaluation that ensues once the diagnosis has been made. The diagnostic methods outlined in. Table 4.1 will be covered in this chapter.

Screening

Historically, the Centers for Disease Control and Prevention (CDC) and the American Association for the Study of Liver Diseases (AASLD) recommend focusingscreening onindividuals with risk factors for hepatitis C and those with an unexplained elevation in aminotransferase levels. Unfortunately, risk based screening has failed to adequately identify identify most individuals with HCV. A recent proposal to the CDC's screening recommendations suggest that all individuals born between 1945 and 1965 get tested once for HCV. 1-time cohort screening is estimated to identify nearly 86% of undiagnosed cases compared with the 21% currently found through risk-based screening (Rein et al., 2012). These individuals are five times more likely to be infected with chronic HCVcompared with other adults and currently account for more than seventy-five percent of infected individuals in the United States. Because HCV is often asymptomatic, it is critical that clinician-sroutinely take an appropriate history in order to identify risk factors, which should be done in combination with appropriate HCV testing and counseling (Alter et al., 2004). The risk factors for hepatitis C were detailed in Chapter 3. For those who test positive during screening, the proposed CDC recommendations call for referral for treatment and a brief screening for alcohol use.

Antibody Testing

Detection of antibodies to the hepatitis C virus is the first step to screen patients in whom HCV is suspected. The presence of HCV antibodies is indicative of either past, current, or resolved infection and cannot discriminate between acute and chronic HCV infection. Antibodies may be detectable as early as 4 to 6 weeks after initial HCV exposure (Fig. 4.1). Development of antibodies may be delayed, however, in patients who have subclinical infection (Beld et al., 1999). Antibodies will persist indefinitely in chronically infected individuals, but anti-HCV titers may decrease and even disappear in patients who clear HCV either spontaneously or after antiviral treatment.

Table 4.1 Diagnostic Testing Used in Patients with Hepatitis C

Basic Laboratory Testing	Complete metabolic panel
	Complete blood count
	Prothrombin time
Serologic Assays	Anti-HCV
	RIBA
Virologic Assays	HCV RNA nucleic acid testing (NAT)
	Quantitative
	Qualitative
	HCV core antigen EIA assay
HCV Genotyping with Subtypes	1a-6
Liver Biopsy	
Noninvasive Markers of Fibrosis	APRI
	FIBROSpect® II
	FibroTest
	HepaScore®
	Transient elastography
Genetic Markers	*IL28B*

©2011, Natasha Walzer, MD

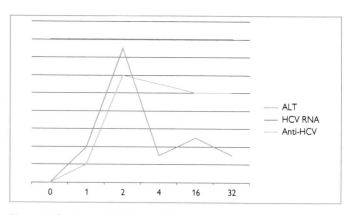

Figure 4.1 Serologic profile of chronic HCV infection (©2011 Natasha Walzer, MD). The ALT will rise within the first month after acute infection and will fluctuate if the disease remains chronic. The HCV RNA will be the earliest detectable evidence for infection and remains fairly constant throughout the course of infection. Anti-HCV will be detectable within 4 to 6 weeks after infection and remains elevated, even if there is clearance of the virus (either through treatment or spontaneously).

The screening test is an enzyme immunoassay (EIA) that detects antibodies to recombinant antigens from core and nonstructural proteins that make up the HCV virion. EIA-2 (second-generation) testing detects HCV antibodies in 95% of infected individuals (Gretch et al., 1993). EIA-3 testing, which adds an additional antigen from the nonstructural region (NS5), has been introduced in many centers across the United States. When compared with second-generation assays, third-generation assays have sensitivities and specificities exceeding 99% and can detect HCV antibodies 2 to 3 weeks earlier (Alborino et al., 2011).

The sensitivity of EIAs appears to be reduced in immunocompromisedpersons, including those on hemodialysis, individuals infected with HIV, and transplant recipients (Lok et al., 1993; Pereir & Levey, 1997; Pereira et al., 1992). Testing for HCV RNA should be considered in immunocompromised patients who are anti-HCV negative but have risk factors for HCV infection and persistently elevated aminotransferase levels.

An over-the-counter testing kit ("Hepatitis C Check" [Home Access Health Corp.]) has been approved by the FDA. The blood sample is obtained at home using a lancet and shipped in a weather-resistant pouch. Upon arrival at the laboratory, standard EIAs are used to test the sample. The sensitivity of this method has been shown to be comparable to hospital-based laboratory testing. Pre- and post-test counseling is available through the manufacturer. In addition, a point-of-care test for rapid detection of anti-HCV was recently approved in Europe. It was shown to be as accurate as laboratory-based testing and could potentially increase access to HCV testing in the community (Lee et al., 2011).

Confirmatory testing using RIBA-2 or RIBA-3 (recombinant immunoblot assay) has been replaced by the direct detection of HCV RNA. It can be used, however, to determine false-positive antibody testing from past infection. Patients who react to two antigens are more likely to have had a past infection than those who react to only one antigen. The sensitivity of the RIBA assay is the same as EIA, but the specificity is increased (Tobler et al., 2000).

CDC recommends that no further testing be performed in an individual who is EIA negative, unless he or she is immunosuppressed. In addition, positive EIA results require confirmatory testing using HCV RNA quantification (Alter et al., 2003).

Patients who test positive for the HCV antibody should have measurement of HCV RNA, using nucleic acid testing (NAT), to confirm active infection and to quantify viremia if treatment is being considered. The presence of HCV RNA can be detected 1 to 3 weeks after infection, approximately 1 month before the appearance of total anti-HCV antibodies. The persistence of HCV RNA after 6 months denotes chronic HCV infection.

Multiple assays are available to detect and quantify viral load using a combination of amplification and detection techniques. Nucleic acid tests are classified into qualitative tests (qualitative polymerase chain reaction [PCR], transcription-mediated amplification [TMA]) and quantitative tests (branched-chain DNA [bDNA] amplification, quantitative PCR, and real-time PCR). Regardless of which method is used, HCV RNA IU/mL is the preferred quantitative unit and has been implemented in most commercial assays. Normalization to international units allows for comparable results among the different assays. Historically, qualitative assays to detect HCV RNA were more sensitive than quantitative assays. However, with the availability of real-time PCR, this is no longer the case. Real-time PCR has a lower limit of detection of 10 to 15 IU/mL and a low false-positive rate. For this reason, real-time PCR has become the method of choice to detect and quantify HCV PCR in clinical practice. Detection of HCV RNA in peripheral blood is used clinically to diagnose chronic HCV infection and to monitor the virologic response to antiviral therapy. A negative NAT result following a positive serologic test result is indicative of a resolved infection. However, low-level viremia can occur during chronic infection, so clinicians should perform a second NAT 6 to 12 months later to confirm the absence of viremia(Scott et al., 2006). In addition, a positive HCV NAT result indicates active infection, regardless of antibody test results.

Routine Laboratory Testing

Measuring the ALT level is an inexpensive but relatively insensitive way to measure disease activity in hepatitis C. Studies have demonstrated a weak association between the ALT measurement and the histopathologic findings on liver biopsy (Inglesby et al., 1999; Marcellin et al., 1997). Approximately 24% to 40% of patients with chronic HCV have normal ALT levels. Once a diagnosis of chronic hepatitis C has been made, measurement of liver enzymes offers little additional clinical information regarding viral activity and fibrosis, although an AST-to-ALT ratio greater than one can be an indicator of cirrhosis.

Thrombocytopenia is often one of the earliest signs of portal hypertension. A complete blood count should be part of the initial evaluation of a patient with hepatitis C. A complete metabolic panel and a PT/INR are also standard tests ordered. A low serum albumin and an elevated INR can reflect the presence of cirrhosis with hepatocellular dysfunction.

HCV Core Antigen Detection

An immunoassay to detect and quantify total HCVcore protein in serum has been developed (Laperche et al., 2003). HCV core antigen levels have an excellent correlation with HCVRNA concentrations and can be considered an alternative to measuring the HCV RNA level (Veillon et al., 2003). Automated testing for antibodies to core protein is less expensive than PCR-based assays. However, core antibody testing has not been adopted in clinical practice because of its relatively low sensitivity, with a lower limit of detection of 20,000 IU/mL.

HCV Genotyping

Hepatitis C is classified into six major genotypes, numbered 1 through 6 with subtypes a–c. The genotypes vary in nucleotide sequence by as much as 30% and subtypes vary by 20%. Seventy-one percent of hepatitis C cases in the United States are infected with HCV genotype 1, including 90% of African Americans. Genotype 2 accounts for 13.5% of all reported HCV cases in the United States, and genotype 3 accounts for 5.5% of the total cases (Lau et al., 1995). The HCV genotype can be determined by direct sequencing from subgenomic regions of the virus, such as core/E1 or NS5B. Historically, genotype was a strong predictor of response to pegylated interferon (PEG-IFN) and ribavirin (RBV) and was used to determine duration of treatment (Lau et al., 1995; Veillon et al., 2003; Yano et al., 1996). The availability of HCV protease inhibitors has led to a paradigm shift. Patients with genotype 1 infection are candidates for therapy with the combination of a protease inhibitor (PI),PEG-IFN, and RBV. The first-generationPIs have a lower barrier to resistance for genotype 1a, resulting in higher sustained response rates for genotype 1b. PEG-IFN and RBV remains the treatment of choice for patients with non-genotype-1 infections, for which the PIs have little or no activity. For these reasons, it is standard to obtain HCV genotyping in any patient who is considering undergoing treatment for hepatitis C.

Liver Biopsy

A liver biopsy is not essential to the diagnosis of chronic hepatitis C and the role of biopsy is evolving as response rates increase and noninvasive tests for hepatic fibrosis improve. Liver biopsy remains the gold standard toquantify inflammation (grade) and fibrosis (stage), which are important in guiding treatment decisions. Biopsy also is useful in identifying concomitant causes of liver disease, as well as documenting the presence of cirrhosis, which has important prognostic and management implications. For example, patientsfound to have cirrhosis on liver biopsy should be started on a surveillance protocol for hepatocellular carcinoma. Sampling error does exist, and specimens shorter than 2 cm can be difficult to interpret.

Liver biopsy findings in a patient with chronic hepatitis C usually consist of a portal lymphocytic infiltrate that may extend and involve the limiting plate. The degree of inflammation and fibrosis can predict the likelihood that a patient will progress to more advanced stages of fibrosis (Yano et al., 1996). For this reason, the AASLD guidelines recommend consideration of antiviral therapy for patients withstage II fibrosis or greater in an effort to prevent development of cirrhosis. Treatment of naïve genotype 1 patients with lesser degrees of fibrosis or without fibrosis staging will likely become common practice now that protease inhibitors provide sustained response rates exceeding 70% for this group (Jacobson et al., 2011; Poordad et al., 2011).

Noninvasive Assessment of Liver Fibrosis

While liver biopsy has been the preferred method to stage hepatitis C, it has several limitations as well asthe risks of pain (20%), bleeding, and hemobilia (0.5%) (Cadranel et al., 2000). Sampling error and intra-observer variability affect the diagnostic accuracy of liver biopsy, even with the use of widely validated histologic scoring systems. As a result, noninvasive diagnosis of liver fibrosis has evolved rapidly over recent years. Fibrosis can be detectedand quantified by assays that measure serum markersand by an imaging technique that detects liver stiffness (transient elastography). The AST-platelet ratio index (APRI) isa validated and widely studied scoring system that is readily available at low cost. It is most effective at excluding significant HCV-related fibrosis (Shaheen& Myers, 2007). It is defined by the following formula: [{AST (IU/l)/ ALT_ULN (IU/L)}× 100]/ platelet count (10^9/L). An APRI less than 0.5 suggests that there is no or minimal fibrosis; an APRI above 1.5 is suggestive of more significant fibrosis. Most scoring systems include a combination of routine laboratory tests with serum biomarkers of fibrosis. Some of these scores have been widely validated in large cohorts of patients (FIBROSpect®II, FibroTest, HepaScore®) (Adams et al., 2005; Cales et al., 2005; Forns et al., 2002; Imbert-Bismut et al., 2001) and are used in clinical practice. The majority of the scoring systems, including the imaging studies,are very accurate in identifying patients with advanced or no fibrosis, but their sensitivity and specificity drop significantly when evaluating for intermediate stages of fibrosis (Parkes et al., 2006). These measurements of liver fibrosis have not been introduced into the practice guidelines as standard of care, but they do have some value in the assessment of liver fibrosis, especially in patients who are not candidates for liver biopsy or as a means of obtaining serial measurements of fibrosis.

Pharmacogenetics Testing

Recent genome-wide association studies have demonstrated a link between a genetic polymorphism near the *IL28B* gene region and response to PEG-IFN-α plus RBV in patients with genotype 1 chronic HCV (Ge et al., 2009; Suppiah et al., 2009; Tanaka et al., 2009). These genetic variations have also been found to be associated with spontaneous clearance of the virus without treatment (Rauch et al., 2010; Thomas et al., 2009). During genetic analysis, the C allele was found to be the strongest established pretreatment predictor of treatment response in HCV genotype 1 patients. Eighty percent of European patients with the C/C genotype cleared the virus, whereas only approximately 30% of those with the T/T genotype did. Interestingly, the favorable genotype was more commonly found in European Americans (39%) compared to African Americans (16%). This may, in part, explain the well-documented difference in response rates between these two groups of patients. Although initially described in genotype 1 patients, a recent study confirms that the presence of C/C genotype also confers an improved response in genotype 2 and 3 patients (Mangia et al., 2010).

IL28B genotyping has multiple potential roles for clinical practice. Patients who have the favorable genotype could be selected to undergo treatment with PEG-IFN with sustained virologic response (SVR) rates comparable to the addition of a PI, but with a reduced cost and side-effect profile. In a retrospective analysis of the REALIZE trial,IL28b genotyping was no longer a predictor of response. Patients with any of the genotypes had response rates exceeding 60%, suggesting that IL28B genotyping may be of limited utility with the addition of telaprevir (Pol et al., 2011). Boceprevir also improved SVR rates in nearly all of the *IL28B* genotype subgroups, with the exception of treatment-naïve patients of the CC genotype (who exhibited high SVR rates regardless of regimen) and previously treated patients with the TT genotype who received response-guided boceprevir plus PEG-IFN/RBV (Poordad et al., 2011).

Conclusion

The decision to screen a patient for hepatitis C should be based on the presence of elevated aminotransferase levels, a risk factor for the acquisition for hepatitis C as stated in the AASLD guidelines, and in accordance with the proposed CDC recommendations, anyone born between from 1945 and 1965. Screening is performed by EIA testing and active infection is confirmed by measuring HCV RNA (Fig. 4.2). Hepatitis C genotype should be determined in potential treatment candidates. Liver biopsy can be performed to stage the liver disease and to assess for other causes of liver injury. Alternatively, noninvasive assays can provide an indication of the degree of fibrosis. Even if a patient is not thought to be an appropriate candidate for treatment of hepatitis C, documenting the presence of cirrhosis or advanced fibrosis has significant health implications, including a risk of liver failure and hepatocellular carcinoma. Proper screening and evaluation of patients with HCV is critical in bringing affected individuals to medical attention so that they can benefit from recent advances in antiviral therapy.

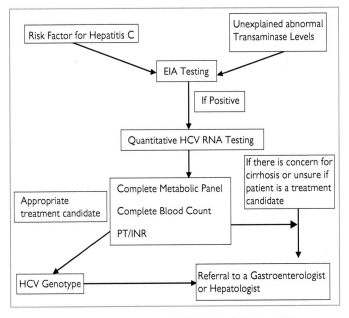

Figure 4.2 Testing algorithm for hepatitis C (©2011, Natasha Walzer, MD)

References

Adams, L. A., M. Bulsara, E. Rossi, et al. (2005). Hepascore: an accurate validated predictor of liver fibrosis in chronic hepatitis C infection. *Clinical Chemistry, 51,* 1867–1873.

Alborino, F., A. Burighel, F. W. Tiller, et al. (2011). Multicenter evaluation of a fully automated third-generation anti-HCV antibody screening test with excellent sensitivity and specificity. *Medical Microbiology and Immunology, 200,* 77–83.

Alter, M. J., W. L. Kuhnert, &L. Finelli (Feb. 7, 2003).Guidelines for laboratory testing and result reporting of antibody to hepatitis C virus. *MMWR Recommendations and Reports.* Available from: http://www.cdc.gov/mmwr/preview/mmwrhtml/rr5203a1.htm

Alter, M. J., L. B. Seeff, B. R. Bacon (2004). Testing for hepatitis C virus infection should be routine for persons at increased risk for infection. *Annals of Internal Medicine, 141,* 715–717.

Beld, M., M. Penning, M. van Putten, et al. (1999). Low levels of hepatitis C virus RNA in serum, plasma, and peripheral blood mononuclear cells of injecting drug users during long antibody-undetectable periods before seroconversion. *Blood, 94,* 1183–1191.

Cadranel, J. F., P. Rufat, & F. Degos (2000). Practices of liver biopsy in France: results of a prospective nationwide survey. For the Group of Epidemiology of the French Association for the Study of the Liver (AFEF). *Hepatology, 32,* 477–481.

Cales, P., F. Oberti, S. Michalak, et al. (2005). A novel panel of blood markers to assess the degree of liver fibrosis. *Hepatology, 42,* 1373–1381.

Centers for Disease Control and Prevention (CDC). *Recommendations for Chronic HCV Infection.* Updated March 20, 2012, Accessed June 13, 2012. http://www.cdc.gov/hepatitis/HCV/GuidelinesC.htm

Forns, X., S. Ampurdanes, J. M. Llovet, et al. (2002). Identification of chronic hepatitis C patients without hepatic fibrosis by a simple predictive model. *Hepatology, 36,* 986–992.

Ge, D., J. Fellay, A. J. Thompson, et al. (2009). Genetic variation in IL28B predicts hepatitis C treatment-induced viral clearance. *Nature, 461,* 399–401.

Gretch, D. R., J. J. Wilson, R. L. Carithers Jr., et al. (1993). Detection of hepatitis C virus RNA: comparison of one-stage polymerase chain reaction (PCR) with nested-set PCR. *Journal of Clinical Microbiology, 31,* 289–291.

Imbert-Bismut, F., V. Ratziu, L. Pieroni, et al. (2001). Biochemical markers of liver fibrosis in patients with hepatitis C virus infection: a prospective study. *Lancet, 357,* 1069–1075.

Inglesby, T. V., R. Rai, J. Astemborski, et al. (1999). A prospective, community-based evaluation of liver enzymes in individuals with hepatitis C after drug use. *Hepatology, 29,* 590–596.

Jacobson, I. M., J. G. McHutchison, G. Dusheiko, et al. (2011). Telaprevir for previously untreated chronic hepatitis C virus infection. *New England Journal of Medicine, 364,* 2405–2416.

Laperche, S., N. Le Marrec, N. Simon, et al. (2003). A new HCV core antigen assay based on disassociation of immune complexes: an alternative to molecular biology in the diagnosis of early HCV infection. *Transfusion, 43,* 958–962.

Lau, J. Y., M. Mizokami, J. A. Kolberg, et al. (1995). Application of six hepatitis C virus genotyping systems to sera from chronic hepatitis C patients in the United States. *Journal of Infectious Diseases, 171,* 281–289.

Lee, S. R., K. W. Kardos, E. Schiff, et al. (2011). Evaluation of a new, rapid test for detecting HCV infection, suitable for use with blood or oral fluid. *Journal of Virological Methods, 172,* 27–31.

Lok, A. S., D. Chien, Q. L. Choo, et al. (1993). Antibody response to core, envelope and nonstructural hepatitis C virus antigens: comparison of immunocompetent and immunosuppressed patients. *Hepatology, 18,* 497–502.

Mangia, A., A. J. Thompson, R. Santoro, et al. (2010). An IL28B polymorphism determines treatment response of hepatitis C virus genotype 2 or 3 patients who do not achieve a rapid virologic response. *Gastroenterology, 139,* 821–827.

Marcellin, P., S. Levy, & S. Erlinger. (1997). Therapy of hepatitis C: patients with normal aminotransferase levels. *Hepatology, 26,* 133S–136S.

Parkes, J., I. N. Guha, P. Roderick, & W. Rosenberg. (2006). Performance of serum marker panels for liver fibrosis in chronic hepatitis C. *Journal of Hepatology, 44,* 462–474.

Pereira, B. J., & A. S. Levey (1997). Hepatitis C virus infection in dialysis and renal transplantation. *Kidney International, 51,* 981–999.

Pereira, B. J., E. L. Milford, R. L. Kirkman, et al. (1992). Prevalence of hepatitis C virus RNA in organ donors positive for hepatitis C antibody and in the recipients of their organs. *New England Journal of Medicine, 327,* 910–915.

Pol, S., J. Aerssens, S. Zeuzem, et al. (2011). *Similar SVR rates in IL28B CC, CT or TT prior relapser, partial- or null-responder patients treated with telaprevir/peginterferon/ribavirin: retrospective analysis of the REALIZE study.* Program and abstracts of the 46th Annual Meeting of the European Association for the Study of the Liver, March 30–April 3, 2011, Berlin, Germany. Abstract 13.

Poordad, F., J-P. Bronowicki, S. C. Gordon, et al. (2011). *IL28B polymorphism predicts virologic response in patients with hepatitis C genotype 1 treated with boceprevir (BOC) combination therapy.* Program and abstracts of the 46th Annual Meeting of the European Association for the Study of the Liver, March 30–April 3, 2011, Berlin, Germany. Abstract 12.

Poordad, F., J. McCone Jr., B. R. Bacon, et al. (2011). Boceprevir for untreated chronic HCV genotype 1 infection. *New England Journal of Medicine, 364,* 1195–1206.

Rauch, A., Z. Kutalik, P. Descombes, et al. (2010). Genetic variation in IL28B is associated with chronic hepatitis C and treatment failure: a genome-wide association study. *Gastroenterology, 138,* 1338–1345.

Rein DB. Smith BD, Wittenborn JS, et al. (2012). The cost-effectiveness of birth-cohort screening for hepatitis C antibody in U.S. primary care settings. *Ann Intern Med, 156(4),* 263–70.

Scott, J. D., B. J. McMahon, D. Bruden, et al. (2006). High rate of spontaneous negativity for hepatitis C virus RNA after establishment of chronic infection in Alaska Natives. *Clinical Infectious Diseases, 42,* 945–952.

Shaheen, A. A., & R. P. Myers (2007). Diagnostic accuracy of the aspartate aminotransferase-to-platelet ratio index for the prediction of hepatitis C-related fibrosis: a systematic review. *Hepatology, 46,* 912–921.

Suppiah, V., M. Moldovan, G. Ahlenstiel, et al. (2009). IL28B is associated with response to chronic hepatitis C interferon-alpha and ribavirin therapy. *Nature Genetics, 41,* 1100–1104.

Tanaka, Y., N. Nishida, M. Sugiyama, et al. (2009). Genome-wide association of IL28B with response to pegylated interferon-alpha and ribavirin therapy for chronic hepatitis C. *Nature Genetics, 41*, 1105–1109.

Thomas, D. L., C. L. Thio, M. P. Martin, et al. (2009). Genetic variation in IL28B and spontaneous clearance of hepatitis C virus. *Nature, 461*, 798–801.

Tobler, L. H., S. R. Lee, S. L. Stramer, et al. (2000). Performance of second- and third-generation RIBAs for confirmation of third-generation HCV EIA-reactive blood donations. Retrovirus Epidemiology Donor Study. *Transfusion, 40*, 917–923.

Veillon, P., C. Payan, G. Picchio, et al. (2003). Comparative evaluation of the total hepatitis C virus core antigen, branched-DNA, and amplicor monitor assays in determining viremia for patients with chronic hepatitis C during interferon plus ribavirin combination therapy. *Journal of Clinical Microbiology, 41*, 3212–3220.

Yano, M., H. Kumada, M. Kage, et al. (1996). The long-term pathological evolution of chronic hepatitis C. *Hepatology, 23*, 1334–1340.

Chapter 5

Pathology of Viral Hepatitis C

Shriram Jakate

Hepatitis C virus (HCV) infection is common worldwide (approximately 3% of the population) and is the leading indication for liver transplantation in the United States (about a third of all cases). Most patients (70% to 90%) who acquire HCV infection develop chronicity, and a significant number of these (20% to 30%) develop cirrhosis and related complications over 10 to 20 years of follow-up. In HCV-related cirrhosis, the annual risk for hepatocellular carcinoma is estimated at 1% to 4% (Lamps & Washington, 2004; Theise et al., 2007). Diagnosis of HCV hepatitis, both acute and chronic, is best made by serologic testing since the microscopic findings are not specific or pathognomonic and immunostaining of liver tissue for HCV is currently not used for diagnostic purposes. Furthermore, infection by any of the various HCV genotypes and subtypes is not associated with individually distinctive histologic characteristics (although genotype 3 has greater predilection for causing steatosis). However, certain histologic changes are consistently observed in acute and chronic HCV hepatitis and features of chronicity and disease progression are best seen microscopically. Thus, pathologic assessment of liver tissue in HCV hepatitis is crucial for the following: (1) determination of the extent of liver injury, including progression to fibrosis and cirrhosis; (2) monitoring response to therapy; and (3) evaluating liver tissue for co-infection or coexistent diseases.

Acute HCV Hepatitis

The term "acute viral hepatitis" is used when hepatic inflammation and elevated serum transaminases levels are present for less than 6 months. Liver biopsy is uncommonly performed in acute viral hepatitis since most cases are either asymptomatic or, in symptomatic patients, the diagnosis is made clinically. When liver tissue is assessed, the histologic abnormalities are not specific but are located predominantly and disproportionately in the lobules rather than portal or periportal areas (the opposite generally occurs in chronic viral hepatitis). The changes are characterized by varying types of necrosis of individual hepatocytes and simultaneous reactive inflammatory and regenerative processes ("necroinflammatory activity"). Scattered individual hepatocytes may show swelling or ballooning degeneration, the lysis of which ("spotty or focal necrosis") provokes collection of small clusters of mononuclear inflammatory cells (lymphocytes and macrophages) and creates disruption in linear cell plate arrangement ("lobular disarray"). Alternatively, hepatocytes may display apoptosis with dense eosinophilic cytoplasm and pyknotic or missing nuclei ("acidophil bodies") with relatively little inflammatory response (Fig. 5.1). The hepatocytic necrosis is often associated with regenerating hepatocytes and hyperplastic Kupffer cells. Occasionally, as part of the hepatocytic injury and inflammatory response, there may be hepatocellular cholestasis with cholangiolar proliferation. None of these features is predictive of predisposition or propensity for future chronicity or disease progression.

Acute HCV Hepatitis with Massive Necrosis and Fulminant Hepatic Failure

Rarely (<1% of cases), acute HCV hepatitis is quite severe and may lead to fulminant hepatic failure. This is associated with high mortality without liver transplantation. Again, the pathologic findings are not diagnostic of viral hepatitis but display sub-massive or massive necrosis similar to other causes, such as drug toxicity or ischemia. Here, instead of necrosis of scattered individual hepatocytes, massive hepatocytic destruction occurs, eliminating and collapsing contiguous large segments of hepatic parenchyma. The surviving hepatocytes attempt brisk regeneration, creating patchy nodularity. If such liver is explanted, it shows a flaccid, collapsed external surface with wrinkling and focal nodularity (Fig. 5.2). Microscopically, the regenerating nodules can be mistaken for cirrhosis. However, unlike cirrhosis, between the regenerating nodules, there

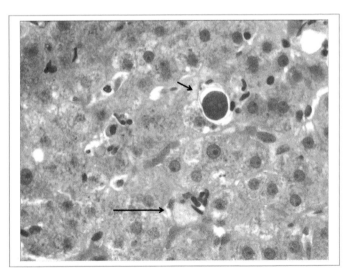

Figure 5.1 Acute HCV hepatitis with ballooned hepatocyte showing spotty necrosis (*long arrow*) and apoptotic acidophil body (*short arrow*). Routine hematoxylin and eosin stain, magnification ×600.

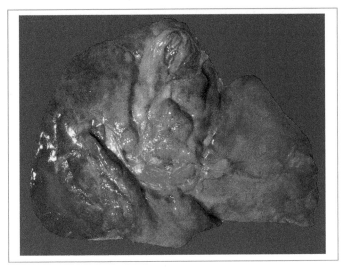

Figure 5.2 Acute HCV hepatitis leading to fulminant hepatic failure and massive necrosis. The external (inferior) surface of the liver shows wrinkled capsule irregular nodularity created by surviving regenerating hepatocytes.

is confluent necrosis with massive loss of hepatocytes and collapsed reticulin framework. The necrosis is associated with severe acute inflammation and prominent bile ductular proliferation with acute cholangiolitis.

Chronic HCV Hepatitis

Chronic HCV hepatitis implies the presence of elevated serum transaminases or hepatic inflammation for over 6 months. As opposed to acute hepatitis, the portal and periportal or interface hepatitis are more predominant or disproportionately greater than lobular changes. The histologic features are not pathognomonic and mimic other forms of chronic hepatitis such as autoimmune hepatitis, drug reactions, and metabolic liver diseases. The portal tracts generally show a dense infiltrate of chronic inflammatory cells, predominantly lymphocytes. This is usually limited to a part of the portal tract ("polar") and adjacent to or surrounding the bile duct ("paraductal or periductal") (Fig. 5.3). Such dense lymphoid aggregate may occasionally show a lymphoid follicle with a germinal center. Other inflammatory cells such as macrophages, plasma cells, and eosinophils are much fewer (if plasma cells or eosinophils are predominant, other diagnoses need to be considered). Periportal areas including the limiting plates often show necroinflammatory activity ("piecemeal necrosis" or "interface hepatitis") (Fig. 5.4). The extent of interface hepatitis is a crucial component of grading of the hepatitis. While every portal tract does not show an equal or uniform level of inflammation, there is general conformity, such that

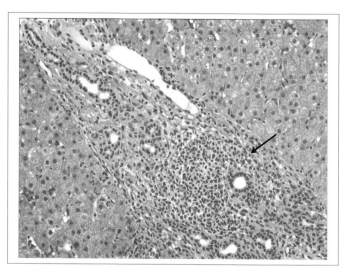

Figure 5.3 Chronic HCV hepatitis showing a lymphoid cell aggregate or nodule restricted to a portion of the portal tract and showing periductal (*arrow*) localization. Routine hematoxylin and eosin stain, magnification ×200.

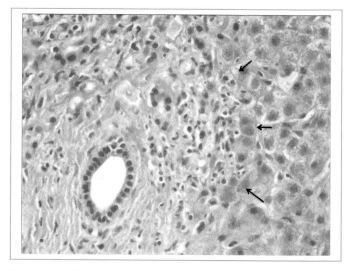

Figure 5.4 Interface hepatitis or piecemeal necrosis showing hepatocytic loss and chronic inflammatory cells at the limiting plate (*arrows*). This is a consistent feature of chronic HCV hepatitis. Routine hematoxylin and eosin stain, magnification ×400.

sampling variation and error is minimized in an adequately sized liver biopsy specimen. The ongoing portal and periportal inflammation eventually results in fibrosis, the progression of which originates in the portal tracts and subsequently involves periportal areas, creates portal–portal (Fig. 5.5) and portal–central fibrous bridges, and leads to diffuse curvilinear fibrosis and cirrhotic nodularity (Fig. 5.6). The lobular inflammation is similar to that seen in acute viral hepatitis, but it is relatively mild and discordant with the portal and interface inflammatory activity. Macrovesicular steatosis is often present, but it is focal and seen in only a few hepatocytes.

Scoring (Grade and Stage) of Chronic HCV Hepatitis

Since most cases of HCV infection lead to chronicity with the potential for end-stage liver disease and hepatic decompensation, it is necessary to monitor the progression of disease as well as the response to therapy. This is done microscopically (unlike the initial diagnosis, which is done serologically). Similar to the grading and staging performed for neoplastic diseases (denoting tumor differentiation and progression), chronic HCV hepatitis is scored for its level of inflammatory activity (grade) and progression to fibrosis (stage). Many different scoring systems for HCV are available. However, it is crucial to adopt a practical scoring system that is consistently applied, easy to follow, and understood and used by the treating physician. The most commonly practiced scoring system employs give categories, each scored 0 to 4 for grade and stage

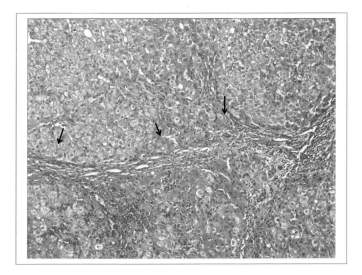

Figure 5.5 Chronic HCV hepatitis showing slender portal–portal bridging fibrosis (*arrows*). Routine hematoxylin and eosin stain, magnification ×100.

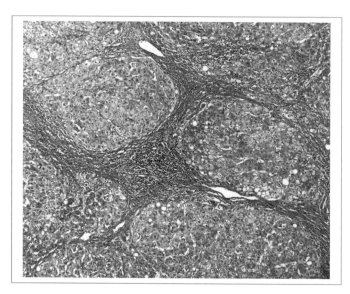

Figure 5.6 HCV hepatitis with cirrhosis showing diffuse curvilinear fibrosis and nodularity. Routine hematoxylin and eosin stain, ×40 magnification.

(Batts & Ludwig, 1995) (Table 5.1). Other systems, such as French Cooperative Study Group (METAVIR) (Bedossa & Poynard, 1996) and Knodell (Knodell et al., 1981), which incorporate more categories and higher total scores, are probably not needed for routine assessment.

Recurrence of HCV Hepatitis in the Graft

New HCV infection after liver transplantation is rare since screening of donated blood products has dramatically decreased post-transfusion infection. However, reinfection of the graft from prior HCV occurs almost universally (except in the few patients who demonstrate sustained virologic response to therapy before transplantation) (Guillouche & Feray, 2011). The re-infection occurs in the same sequence as it does before transplantation. In the early post-transplantation period, there is (frequently asymptomatic) acute HCV hepatitis. In a few patients (<5%), there is severe fulminant-like acute hepatitis designated as "fibrosing cholestatic hepatitis," which occurs in the setting of immunosuppression and may rapidly lead to graft failure. More than 70% of patients develop chronic hepatitis and 10% to 50% cirrhosis in 5 years. Recurrent HCV is more aggressive in the graft than in the original native liver, likely due to the transplantation-related immunosuppression. Histologic diagnosis of recurrent HCV is made more challenging in the graft due to potential

Table 5.1 Scoring System for Grading Inflammation and Staging Fibrosis

	Portal/Periportal Inflammation	Lobular Inflammation
Grade 0	None	None
Grade 1	Portal inflammation only	Minimal inflammatory cells but no hepatocellular death
Grade 2	Mild interface hepatitis	Mild inflammation with focal cell death
Grade 3	Moderate interface hepatitis	Moderate with hepatocellular degeneration
Grade 4	Severe interface hepatitis	Severe with prominent diffuse hepatocellular damage

Scoring System for Staging

Stage 0	No fibrosis
Stage 1	Fibrous portal expansion, confined to enlarged portal tracts
Stage 2	Periportal expansion, rare portal–portal fibrous septa
Stage 3	Bridging fibrosis with architectural distortion but no obvious cirrhosis
Stage 4	Definite cirrhosis

graft-related considerations such as rejection and hepatitis related to drug toxicity or perfusion deficit.

HCV and Co-infection by Other Viruses

HCV and HBV

Dual infection by HCV and HBV may occur due to their similar modes of transmission and high prevalence in endemic areas and high-risk populations (Chu et al., 2008). Overall, HCV coexists in 5% to 20% of patients with HBV hepatitis. Rather than simultaneous infection, the most common sequence is HCV superinfection in HBV-infected patients. Such patients may show higher rates of fulminant hepatic failure, cirrhosis, and hepatocellular carcinoma than with HCV infection alone. Histologically, the chronic hepatitis may show mixed features of HCV and HBV (including reactive hepatocytic anisonucleosis, ground-glass cytoplasm, sanded nuclei, and positive immunostaining for HBsAg and HBcAg).

HCV and HIV

The prevalence of HCV in HIV co-infection varies in different high-risk groups, but it is highest among injection drug users (72% to 95%) (Operskalski & Kovacs, 2011). The impact of HCV on HIV disease progression is debatable, but HIV has a negative impact on natural progression of HCV, including persistence of high viral load and more rapid progression to cirrhosis and hepatic decompensation. Histologically, patients co-infected with HIV and HCV show no additional features other than HCV-related changes.

HCV and Coexistent Liver Diseases

HCV and Autoimmune Hepatitis

Both acute and chronic HCV and autoimmune hepatitis (AIH) can histologically mimic each other. Their distinction is vital given the potentially differing disease progressions and divergent and conflicting therapeutic choices. The histologic suspicion of AIH is enhanced if there are prominent interface plasma cells and rosettes (Badiani et al., 2010) and noticeable lymphocytes in the sinusoidal spaces. Even with these histologic pointers, coexistence of AIH is uncommon in HCV and serologic correlation with elevated autoantibodies and gamma globulin levels is needed for the diagnosis of AIH.

HCV and Nonalcoholic Fatty Liver Disease (NAFLD)

HCV and NAFLD are both very common in the population and often coexist, and each may adversely influence the severity of the other (Younossi & McCullough, 2009). The presence of a few hepatocytes showing incidental macrovesicular steatosis is common in HCV, but diffuse macrovesicular steatosis coupled with other findings of NAFLD such as ballooning, steatohepatitis, and prominent hepatocytic nuclear glycogen suggests coexistent NAFLD.

HCV and EtOH Hepatitis

Coexistence of HCV and EtOH hepatitis may occur and is identified clinically, serologically, and histologically (Goldar-Najafi et al., 2002). Apart from HCV-related findings, there may be prominent macrovesicular steatosis, ballooning, Mallory bodies, neutrophilic inflammatory response, and perivenular fibrosis suggestive of EtOH.

References

Badiani, R. G., V. Becker, R. M. Perez, et al. (2010). Is autoimmune hepatitis a frequent finding among HCV patients with intense interface hepatitis? *World Journal of Gastroenterology, 16*(29), 3704–3708.

Batts, K. P., & J. Ludwig (1995). Chronic hepatitis: An update on terminology and reporting. *American Journal of Surgical Pathology, 19*, 1409–1417.

Bedossa, P., & T. Poynard (1996). An algorithm for the grading of activity in chronic hepatitis C. *Hepatology, 24*, 289–293.

Chu, C-J., & S-D. Lee (2008). Hepatitis B virus/hepatitis C virus coinfection: Epidemiology, clinical features, viral interactions and treatment. *Journal of Gastroenterology and Hepatology, 23*, 512–520.

Goldar-Najafi, A., F. D. Gordon, W. D. Lewis, et al. (2002). Liver transplantation for alcoholic liver disease with or without hepatitis C. *International Journal of Surgical Pathology, 10*(2), 115–122.

Guillouche, P., & C. Feray (2011). Systematic review: anti-viral therapy of recurrent hepatitis C after liver transplantation. *Alimentary Pharmacology & Therapeutics, 33*, 163–174.

Knodell, R., K. Ishak, W. Black, et al. (1981). Formulation and application of a numerical scoring system for assessing histological activity in asymptomatic chronic active hepatitis. *Hepatology, 1,* 431–435.

Lamps, L. W., & K. Washington (2004). Acute and chronic hepatitis. In: R. D. Odze, J. R. Goldblum, & J. M. Crawford (Eds.), *Surgical pathology of the GI tract, liver, biliary tract and pancreas* (pp. 783–810). Saunders.

Operskalski, E. A., & A. Kovacs (2011). HIV/HCV co-infection: Pathogenesis, clinical complications, treatment and new therapeutic technologies. *Current HIV/AIDS Reports, 8,* 12–22.

Theise, N. D., H. C. Bodenheimer, & L. D. Ferrell (2007). Acute and chronic viral hepatitis. In: A. D. Burt, B. C. Portman, & L. D. Ferrell (Eds.), *MacSween's pathology of the liver* (pp. 399–441). Churchill Livingstone Elsevier.

Younossi, Z. M., & A. J. McCullough (2009). Metabolic syndrome, non-alcoholic fatty liver disease and hepatitis C virus: impact on disease progression and treatment response. *Liver International, 29*(s2), 3–12.

Chapter 6

Acute Hepatitis C

Christin N. Price and Arthur Y. Kim

The majority of HCV infections in the United States occurred during the 1970s and 1980s (see Chapter 2, Epidemiology), but a new epidemic of HCV is occurring primarily related to a resurgence of injection drug use (IDU) in certain parts of the country. In addition to injection drug users, an increasingly recognized group at risk for acute HCV is men who have sex with men (MSM), particularly those with preexisting HIV infection. Since the vast majority of HCV infections are asymptomatic, detecting an early-stage infection is a clinical challenge. The identification of acute HCV requires knowledge of behavioral risk factors and proper interpretation of diagnostic tests. It is especially important to identify acute HCV because treatment during the acute stage of HCV infection (particularly in the first 6 months) is associated with better outcomes than treatment during the chronic stage.

Definition

While definitions vary in the literature, acute hepatitis C infection can be defined as the first 6 months after infection. It is during this period when spontaneous clearance of virus may occur and the efficacy of early antiviral treatments is maximal. Figure 6.1 displays the natural history of acute HCV for both those who spontaneously clear infection and those who develop persistent or chronic infection (Fig. 6.1).

Incidence

After the implementation of blood-product screening for HCV infection and a decrease in IDU rates, the incidence of acute hepatitis C infection declined after peaking in 1992. This decline continued until 2005, when levels reached a plateau (CDC, 2011a). According to the CDC's National Notifiable Disease Surveillance System, the overall national rate of acute HCV infection is 0.3 cases per 100,000 population, and in 2007, 849 cases of acute hepatitis C were confirmed by this system. However, after accounting for asymptomatic infection (the vast majority of acute cases), lack of presentation to medical care, and underreporting, the estimated incidence of acute HCV infection was 17,000 cases nationwide in 2007 (Daniels et al., 2009).

More recently, there has been a concerning rise in rates of HCV infection among young individuals in certain regions of the United States. Between 2002

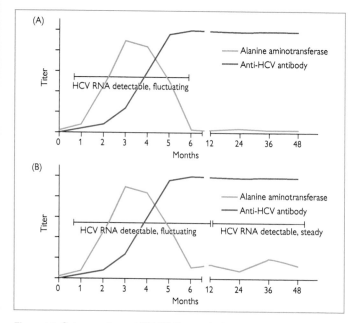

Figure 6.1 Outcomes of acute HCV. (A) Course of HCV infection and spontaneous resolution. (B) Course of HCV infection and progression to chronic infection. Key points include the appearance of HCV RNA prior to ALT elevation and development of antibody and that the acute infection period includes HCV RNA fluctuations that often exceed 1 log.

and 2009, there was an increase in reported acute HCV infections among 15- to 24-year-olds in Massachusetts from 65 to 113 cases per 100,000 population. In response, the Massachusetts Department of Public Health launched a surveillance program from 2007 to 2009 further examining and characterizing the risk factors in this age group. IDU was definitively the most common risk factor for new HCV infection. Of those cases where risk factors were reported (1,196), 72% reported previous or current IDU, and of these, 84% reported injecting drugs within the 12 months prior to becoming infected (CDC, 2011a).

Historically, HCV infection rates have been higher among males in all age groups. However, the male-to-female ratio of acute infection rates has been declining since 2002, and in 2008, the CDC reported for the first time that acute HCV infection rates were equal (0.3 cases per 100,000 population) between males and females.

With respect to race and ethnicity, acute HCV infection rates had been highest among American Indian/Alaskan natives and blacks, with lower rates occurring among Caucasians and Hispanics during the initial epidemic in the 1970s and 1980s. In contrast, in the surveillance report from Massachusetts, the majority of acute HCV infections that were reported between 2007 and 2009 occurred in whites (78%) compared to Hispanics (8%), blacks (3%), and Asians

(2%), signaling a shift in IDU behaviors by ethnicity (Broz & Ouellet, 2008; CDC, 2011a).

There has also been an increase in sexually acquired acute HCV infection among MSM, especially in HIV-infected MSM (Vogel et al., 2011).

Other potential routes of transmission leading to acute HCV include nosocomial (exposure to contaminated needles, syringes, or multi-use vials), occupational (via needlesticks), unsafe tattoos, and intranasal cocaine. Household transmission is extremely rare and may involve sharing of razors or toothbrushes (see Chapter 2, Epidemiology).

Clinical Features

The majority of acute HCV infections are asymptomatic. Of the 20% to 30% of patients who become symptomatic with acute HCV infection, the most common symptoms are nonspecific and include fatigue, myalgias, right upper quadrant abdominal pain, nausea/vomiting, and poor appetite. Only 10% to 20% of patients experience clinical evidence of hepatitis (elevated alanine aminotransferase >10 times the upper limit of normal) and jaundice (Maheshwari et al., 2008). In the minority of cases that are symptomatic, acute hepatitis occurs 2 to 12 weeks after the exposure and can last an additional 2 to 12 weeks. Acute HCV infection rarely progresses to fulminant liver failure. Extrahepatic manifestations of chronic hepatitis C infection such as vasculitis, cryoglobulinemia, porphyria cutanea tarda, and membranous glomerulonephritis are not associated with acute infection (Maheshwari et al., 2008).

It is during this period when individuals may still spontaneously clear the virus on their own (approximately 20% of those infected). However, the remainder develop chronic HCV infection and of these, up to 20% will develop cirrhosis and other complications of liver disease (see Chapter 3, Natural History).

Diagnosis

The diagnosis of acute HCV infection is a clinical one based on risk factors, known exposures, and symptoms followed by confirmatory testing (Table 6.1).

History

The fact that 85% to 90% of cases of acute hepatitis C infection are asymptomatic makes assessment for behavioral risk factors crucial to identify acute HCV infection. High-risk groups are listed in Table 6.2. The most common risk factor for acquiring acute HCV remains IDU. The incidence of HCV infection is between 20 and 40 infections per 100 person-years in those who inject drugs. The timing of *initiation* of injecting drugs is crucial to determining an individual's risk for acquiring new HCV infection because the highest rates are among individuals who have started within the past 12 months (Hagan et al., 2008). Likewise, a detailed history of *habits* while using intravenous drugs includes understanding the number of sharing partners and the timing of sharing of needles

Table 6.1 Diagnosis of Acute HCV

Definite

Seroconversion (positive anti-HCV antibody with negative HCV in the past year)

Seronegative window (HCV RNA positive with negative anti-HCV antibody, subsequent seroconversion)

Probable

History of recent high-risk exposures and/or recent illness consistent with acute HCV

Supporting data:

Elevated liver chemistry test results in absence of other causes

HCV antibody positive

HCV RNA fluctuations >1.0 log

HCV RNA <10^5 IU/mL

Spontaneous clearance of HCV

and syringes. While intravenous drug users may not share needles and syringes, sharing of other drug paraphernalia (e.g., cookers, cottons, water) is relatively common and has been associated with a threefold higher rate of seroconversion compared with those who share no paraphernalia (Hagan et al., 2011). Among persons who do not inject drugs, there is little evidence for specific screening after activities that theoretically expose a person to infected blood, such as body piercing and tattoos.

Among MSM, a detailed sexual history is warranted, with particular attention to sexual practices that would lead to mucosal damage (e.g., use of dilative sex toys), use of phosphodiesterase 5 inhibitors, illicit drug use during sex, sex causing anal bleeding, and group sex, as these were found to be associated with increased rates of acute HCV acquisition (CDC, 2011b; Vogel et al., 2011).

A barrier to ascertaining risk factors for acute HCV is the underreporting of these behaviors to providers, due to associated stigma.

Symptoms and Signs

Most patients are asymptomatic or minimally symptomatic from acute HCV. Some may report a flu-like illness, with or without jaundice in the weeks prior to presentation; such history increases clinical suspicion for acute HCV but by itself is not diagnostic. On physical exam, jaundice may or may not be present and there may be stigmata of other comorbidities (i.e., scars and infections of the skin associated with IDU), but the physical exam would most often be unrevealing or nonspecific.

Diagnostic Testing

Specific tests are covered in Chapter 4, Diagnostic Testing; below is a guide on how to interpret these tests in the context of acute HCV.

Antibody Testing

The definitive way to diagnose new HCV infection is to document seroconversion in a person with previously seronegative status. Unfortunately, HCV antibodies alone are not an ideal measure of acute infection since they can remain undetectable for several weeks after initial infection and are therefore insensitive immediately following infection. Development of antibodies titers is further delayed in HIV-positive MSM, with a median time to seroconversion of 3 months (Thomson et al., 2009).

Past testing may be absent or results uncertain, especially as the care of injection drug users is often fragmented. Moreover, a positive antibody is not specific for acute infection, as they remain elevated throughout the course of infection. Thus, a single positive antibody test is not diagnostic of acute HCV alone without additional supporting data from the history and other laboratory testing.

Aminotransferases and Bilirubin

Acute hepatitis is an indication for further evaluation, especially when risk factors are present. Elevations of alanine aminotransferase (ALT) are greater than aspartate aminotransferase (AST), and a cholestatic picture is rarely encountered. Jaundice and hyperbilirubinemia may accompany severe elevations of ALT in a small minority of cases. Seroconversion has been documented with minimal changes in liver function tests during the acute phase and can be transiently within normal range; thus, the absence of elevations does not exclude acute HCV infection. As the diagnosis of acute HCV needs to be timely to provide maximal treatment benefits, rapid follow-up of elevated liver function tests is recommended even if the patient is asymptomatic.

Viral Load Testing

HCV RNA may be detectable as early as 1 to 2 weeks after infection at times followed by a sharp rise in ALT levels. Therefore, a detectable HCV RNA with absence of anti-HCV antibodies (during the "seronegative window") is strongly suggestive of acute infection.

Both low viral titers (1 log) may be present during acute infection and are not common during the later phases of HCV infection (McGovern et al., 2009). Serial HCV RNA testing may be helpful to support a diagnosis of acute HCV and also to determine outcome (spontaneous clearance vs. persistence). Spontaneous clearance is also rare in the chronic phase of infection and suggests that the patient is in the acute phase.

HCV RNA can help diagnose reinfection after viral clearance (as antibodies are already elevated from the first infection).

Other Testing

As acute HCV infection may be difficult to distinguish from other causes of acute hepatitis (especially when added to chronic HCV infection where both HCV antibody and HCV RNA may be positive), tests for other causes of enzyme elevation are recommended (e.g., anti-HAV IgM, HBVSAg, and anti-HBV core IgM, abdominal ultrasound). If the patient is viremic and qualifies as a candidate for antiviral treatment, a HCV genotype is recommended. Recently, genetic polymorphisms related to interleukin-28B (beta subunit of IL-28, or interferon-lambda-3) have been linked to both spontaneous and treatment-induced clearance. While this genetic test may help with prognosis, its utility in the acute setting has yet to be determined.

Treatment

There are no standard guidelines regarding treatment of acute HCV, and the published data are variable. Many studies have shown that treatment of acute HCV infection with courses that are shorter and less intense than those used during chronic infection is highly effective (Maheshwari et al., 2008).

Because *symptomatic* acute HCV infection seems to be associated with a higher rate of spontaneous clearance of HCV, some authorities suggest waiting a certain amount of time before initiating treatment. Waiting up to 12 weeks in symptomatic patients to see if they clear the virus spontaneously before starting treatment is cost-effective, avoids unnecessary treatment for individuals who spontaneously clear HCV, and is associated with sustained virologic response (SVR) on par with those starting treatment immediately (Maheshwari et al., 2008). For asymptomatic individuals, however, there are no clear data available to suggest the optimal timing of treatment initiation. Since these individuals are less likely to clear the virus spontaneously, some authorities recommend immediate therapy.

There is also considerable debate as to the optimal regimen to treat acute HCV infection. Standard interferon treatment has clearance rates as high as 98% with only 24 weeks of treatment (Jaeckel et al., 2001). Pegylated interferon (PEG-IFN) is easier to administer and has comparable efficacy to standard interferon so is now commonly used. While there are no head-to-head comparisons, regimens including PEG-IFN α-2a and PEG-IFN α-2b showed high SVR rates (Corey et al., 2010). Combination therapy with PEG-IFN and ribavirin has proven benefit in chronic HCV infection, but to date there are no randomized clinical trials comparing monotherapy versus combination therapy for acute HCV. Existing data suggest that combination therapy is well tolerated and has similar SVR rates to monotherapy (Ghany et al., 2009). Novel protease inhibitors have not been studied in acute HCV infection.

In HIV-negative individuals, a duration of treatment of at least 12 weeks produces acceptable SVR rates that are not significantly different from SVR rates of 24 weeks of treatment. Increased side effects and treatment discontinuation are, however, seen more often with longer treatment duration. The American Association for the Study of Liver Diseases (AASLD) guidelines state that a minimum of 12 weeks of treatment is reasonable and up to 24 weeks of therapy can be considered (Ghany et al., 2009). HIV-positive individuals with acute HCV are typically treated for 24 to 48 weeks (Vogel et al., 2011). Those who achieve a rapid virologic response (RNA negative at week 4) are the best candidates for shortened antiviral therapy.

Prevention

There is no currently available vaccine for the prevention of acute HCV infection. HCV seroconversion rates have declined in injection drug users over the past decades, suggesting that HCV is preventable (Hagan et al., 2008). Preventive measures incorporate education and counseling regarding risk reduction, substance abuse treatment including opiate replacement therapy, and needle exchange programs for those actively injecting. Programs with multiple components appear to be the most effective at reducing the incidence of HCV infection (Hagan et al., 2011). Those with either spontaneous or treatment-induced clearance should be counseled to reduce risk behaviors for reacquisition and evaluated regularly for the possibility of reinfection.

References

Broz, D., & L. J. Ouellet (2008). Racial and ethnic changes in heroin injection in the United States: implications for the HIV/AIDS epidemic. *Drug & Alcohol Dependence, 94*(1-3), 221–233.

CDC (2011a). Hepatitis C virus infection among adolescents and young adults— Massachusetts, 2002–2009. *MMWR Morbidity & Mortality Weekly Reports, 60*(17), 537–541.

CDC (2011b). Sexual transmission of hepatitis C virus among HIV-infected men who have sex with men—New York City, 2005–2010. *MMWR Morbidity & Mortality Weekly Reports, 60*, 945–950.

Corey, K. E., J. Mendez-Navarro, E. C. Gorospe, H. Zheng, & R. T. Chung (2010). Early treatment improves outcomes in acute hepatitis C virus infection: a meta-analysis. *Journal of Viral Hepatitis, 17*(3), 201–207.

Daniels, D., S. Grytdal, & A. Wasley (2009). Surveillance for acute viral hepatitis— United States, 2007. *MMWR Surveillance Summary, 58*(3), 1–27.

Ghany, M. G., D. B. Strader, D. L. Thomas, & L. B. Seeff (2009). Diagnosis, management, and treatment of hepatitis C: an update. *Hepatology, 49*(4), 1335–1374.

Hagan, H., E. R. Pouget, D. C. Des Jarlais, & C. Lelutiu-Weinberger (2008). Meta-regression of hepatitis C virus infection in relation to time since onset of illicit drug injection: the influence of time and place. *American Journal of Epidemiology, 168*(10), 1099–1109.

Hagan, H., E. R. Pouget, & D. C. Des Jarlais (2011). A systematic review and meta-analysis of interventions to prevent hepatitis C virus infection in people who inject drugs. *Journal of Infectious Diseases, 204*(1), 74–83.

Jaeckel, E., M. Cornberg, H. Wedemeyer, et al. (2001). Treatment of acute hepatitis C with interferon alfa-2b. *New England Journal of Medicine, 345*(20), 1452–1457.

Maheshwari, A., S. Ray, & P. J. Thuluvath (2008). Acute hepatitis C. *Lancet, 372*(9635), 321–332.

McGovern, B. H., C. E. Birch, M. J. Bowen, et al. (2009). Improving the diagnosis of acute hepatitis C virus infection with expanded viral load criteria. *Clinical Infectious Diseases 49*(7), 1051–1060.

Thomson, E. C., E. Nastouli, J. Main, et al. (2009). Delayed anti-HCV antibody response in HIV-positive men acutely infected with HCV. *AIDS, 23*(1), 89–93.

Vogel, M., C. Boesecke, & J. K. Rockstroh (2011). Acute hepatitis C infection in HIV-positive patients. *Current Opinion Infectious Diseases, 24*(1), 1–6.

Chapter 7

Chronic Hepatitis C

Rohit Satoskar

Scope of the Problem

Hepatitis C remains a global problem. It is estimated that the worldwide prevalence of HCV is as high as 3%, or 170 million individuals. Prevalence estimates vary by region and are highest in Africa and the Eastern Mediterranean region. An estimated 14 million people in the Americas and 83 million people in Asia have chronic HCV. In the United States, the Centers for Disease Control and Prevention (CDC) estimate that 3.2 million people are chronically infected with HCV. The majority of these cases are those born between 1945 and 1965 who were infected during the 1970s and 1980s when infection rates were the highest. Prevalence of chronic hepatitis C is directly related to the previous incidence of acute hepatitis C. This varies depending on age and time. Fortunately, in the United States, the incidence of acute hepatitis C appears to be decreasing: in 2008, only 878 cases of acute HCV infection were reported to the CDC. Because most cases of acute HCV are asymptomatic, this is likely an underrepresentation of the estimated 18,000 cases. Despite decreases in the incidence of acute infection, as the duration of infection in those with chronic HCV increases, the incidences of cirrhosis, decompensation, hepatocellular carcinoma (HCC), and liver-related deaths are expected to increase over the next decade (Fig. 7.1).

Presentation

The clinical presentation of chronic HCV depends largely on the stage of the underlying liver disease. There may be a wide range of presentations, from asymptomatic patients found to have abnormal ALT levels, to those who present with decompensated liver cirrhosis.

Symptoms

The majority of patients found to have chronic hepatitis C do not exhibit specific symptoms. Of those with symptoms, the most common complaint is fatigue. Additional symptoms may include nausea, weight loss, arthralgias, or weakness. Less commonly, patients may present with extrahepatic manifestations of chronic HCV such as arthritis, renal dysfunction, autoimmune disorders, lichen planus, porphyria cutanea tarda, or leukocytoclastic vasculitis (Table 7.1).

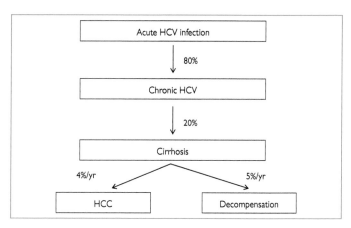

Figure 7.1 Natural history of HCV infection

Table 7.1 Chronic HCV, Extrahepatic Manifestations/Associations
Dermatologic
Lichen planus
Porphyria cutanea tarda
Leukocytoclastic vasculitits
Raynaud's phenomenon
Rheumatologic
Arthritis/arthralgia
Myalgia
Hematologic
Essential mixed cryoglobulinemia
Monoclonal gammopathy
Lymphoma
Renal
Membranoproliferative nephritis
Other
Sicca syndrome
Uveitis
Neuropathy
Diabetes mellitus

Laboratory Abnormalities

A positive anti-HCV antibody by second- or third-generation enzyme-linked immunosorbent assay (ELISA) has a greater than 90% positive predictive value in high-prevalence populations. Patients with a positive HCV antibody should undergo confirmatory testing of HCV infection. Most commonly, testing for serum HCV RNA detection by polymerase chain reaction (PCR) is performed. Patients who are immunocompromised or with end-stage renal disease on dialysis may not exhibit HCV antibodies even in the setting of chronic infection. In these populations, patients at risk should be tested for serum HCV RNA even in the absence of a positive HCV antibody test.

Differentiation between acute and chronic infection must be made on the basis of clinical presentation. Patients with a recent known exposure to HCV, high ALT level, clinical symptoms of acute hepatitis, and known previous normal ALT results should be considered for the possibility of acute HCV. The remainder of patients will likely have chronic HCV.

Two thirds of patients with chronic HCV will exhibit an elevated ALT reading. The degree of elevation in ALT tends to vary over time. ALT levels do not correlate well with the severity of liver histology. HCV genotyping should be performed in all patients with chronic HCV who are considered for therapy.

Cirrhosis

The majority of morbidity and mortality in patients with chronic HCV results from the development of cirrhosis of the liver. Approximately 80% of patients with acute HCV infection will develop chronic disease. Age at infection may influence the progression to chronic disease, with younger patients more likely to clear acute HCV. Of the patients who develop chronic hepatitis C, up to 20% will eventually progress to cirrhosis of the liver. In general, progression of disease occurs slowly, with a median time of 30 years for development of cirrhosis. Factors associated with increased rates of fibrosis include longer duration of infection, alcohol consumption, age over 40 years at infection, male gender, elevated ALT level, and co-infection with HIV (Table 7.2).

Once cirrhosis has developed, if well compensated, 5-year survival ranges from 83% to 91%. Decompensated disease (defined as ascites, hepatic encephalopathy, impaired hepatic synthetic function, or variceal bleeding) may occur at a rate of up to 5% per year. Ascites is generally the most common presenting form of decompensation. Unfortunately, after decompensation, 5-year survival drops to 28% to 50%. Due to poor spontaneous survival rates, patients with decompensated cirrhosis should be considered for liver transplantation.

Table 7.2 Risk Factors for Increased Fibrosis in Chronic HCV
Longer duration of infection
Alcohol consumption >50 g/day
Age >40 years at infection
Male gender
HIV co-infection
Steatosis

In general, the complications of cirrhosis can be divided in those due to portal hypertension and those due to liver insufficiency or decreased synthetic dysfunction. Varices, variceal bleeding, ascites, spontaneous bacterial peritonitis, and hepatorenal syndrome are direct results of portal hypertension. Hepatic encephalopathy results from a combination of portal hypertension and impaired liver function. Other complications of cirrhosis include HCC and the liver–lung syndromes: hepatopulmonary syndrome and portopulmonary hypertension (Table 7.3).

Varices and Variceal Bleeding

Up to 50% of cirrhotic patients will have gastroesophageal varices at diagnosis. The prevalence of varices increases with the severity of underlying liver disease according to Child-Pugh score. Greater than 75% of patients who present with Child C cirrhosis will have gastroesophageal varices. Short-term mortality from acute variceal hemorrhage, while improved over the past two decades, remains high at about 30%. Because of the prevalence of varices in cirrhosis and the high risk of mortality associated with variceal bleeding, it is recommended that all patients undergo screening for varices with upper endoscopy. If present, the size of varices at endoscopy is one of the greatest predictors of future bleeding. Patients with large esophageal varices have a 30% risk of bleeding over 2 years. These patients should undergo primary prophylaxis of bleeding with a nonselective beta blocker or with serial endoscopic variceal ligation (EVL).

Hepatocellular Carcinoma

HCC is the fifth most common solid tumor worldwide and accounts for 5.6% of all cancers. The incidence of HCC has been rising since the early 1980s, and it is now the third leading cause of cancer-related mortality. There is significant geographic variation in the incidence of HCC, with highest rates in Asia and sub-Saharan Africa. Recently, the incidence of HCC in the United States has been on the rise, likely secondary to chronic HCV infection. Eighty percent of HCC cases occur in patients with underlying cirrhosis of the liver.

Overall, chronic HCV infection accounts for up to 20% of HCC cases. The yearly incidence of HCC in patients with cirrhosis from all causes is 2% to 8%.

Table 7.3 Complications of Cirrhosis
Variceal bleeding
Ascites
Spontaneous bacterial peritonitis
Jaundice
Hepatorenal syndrome
Hepatocellular carcinoma (HCC)
Hepatopulmonary syndrome
Portopulmonary hypertension
Hepatic encephalopathy
Protein-calorie malnutrition

While most cases of HCC in patients with chronic HCV occur in the setting of cirrhosis, there are also documented cases of HCC development in HCV patients without cirrhosis. Data from HALT-C showed that this 5-year cumulative risk of developing HCC with bridging fibrosis was 4.1%. Patients with chronic HCV and co-infection with HBV or HIV are at increased risk of HCC. Those with HCV/HIV co-infection may have a 10- to 20-fold increased risk of HCC. Chronic HCV patients with porphyria cutanea tarda and alcohol consumption are also at increased risk of HCC. Recent data suggest that patients with chronic HCV who achieve a sustained virologic response (SVR) with treatment reduce their risk of developing HCC.

Screening and Surveillance

Screening for cancers has now become routine practice in medicine. Screening is a public health service in which members of a defined population are offered a test to identify individuals who are likely to benefit from further testing or treatment aimed at reducing the risk of a disease or its complications. Surveillance, on the other hand, is the continuous monitoring of disease occurrence using the screening test within an at-risk population to achieve the same goals as screening. The utility of screening high-risk populations for HCC has been debated for many years, largely due to the lack of multiple randomized controlled trials. However, surveillance is widely accepted and applied.

According to the American Association for the Study of Liver Diseases (AASLD) guidelines, patients with underlying cirrhosis from chronic HCV should undergo surveillance for HCC with ultrasound every 6 months (Table 7.4). Ultrasound has a sensitivity between 65% and 94% and a specificity of more than 90% when used for screening. The use of ultrasound has been criticized due to operator dependence and difficult visualization in patients who are obese. CT and MRI have demonstrated excellent specificity when used for diagnosis but have not been well studied in the setting of surveillance. While many centers use CT or MRI to screen for HCC, it is also not clear that this approach is cost-effective. The use of tumor markers, including alpha fetoprotein (AFP), Des-gamma-carboxy prothrombin (DCP), and prothrombin induced by vitamin K absence II (PIVKA II), has recently been omitted from the AASLD practice guidelines due to the lack of strong data to support this practice. Despite this, other societies continue to recommend the use of tumor markers, and many U.S. centers continue to test for them.

While there are no current recommendations to screen patients with chronic HCV and stage 3 fibrosis, many centers will do so due to the increased

Table 7.4 Recommendations for HCC Surveillance in High-Risk Patients			
American Association for the Study of Liver Diseases (AASLD)	European Association for the Study of the Liver (EASL)	Asian Pacific Association for the Study of the Liver (APASL)	National Comprehensive Cancer Network (NCCN)
Ultrasound every 6 months	Ultrasound and AFP every 6 months	Ultrasound and AFP every 6 months	Ultrasound and AFP every 6 months

risk of HCC as shown in the HALT-C studies, as well as the possibility of understaging with biopsy. Screening at more frequent intervals (i.e., 3 months) has not been shown to be more effective.

Standard recall procedures should be in place for those found to have an abnormality on screening. Patients with an abnormality on screening ultrasound should have evaluation with a four-phase dynamic MRI or CT to more definitively characterize the lesion. If the findings are characteristic of HCC on either study, the lesion should be managed as such. If atypical on both studies, biopsy may be considered to reach a definitive diagnosis.

Various therapies are available for the treatment of HCC. Treatment should be pursued in conjunction with a liver transplant center or a care provider experienced in the management of HCC. Choice of treatment depends on the degree of underlying liver disease, stage of HCC, comorbidities, and patient preference. For early HCC, "curative" measures such as liver transplantation and hepatic resection may be considered. Transarterial chemoembolization (TACE), radiofrequency ablation (RFA), and other locoregional therapies may be considered in patients who are not surgical candidates. For patients with advanced disease, systemic chemotherapy such as sorafenib may be considered.

References

El-Serag, H. B., H. Hampel, C. Yeh, & L. Rabeneck (2002). Extrahepatic manifestations of hepatitis C among United States male veterans. *Hepatology, 36*(6), 1439–1445.

Fattovich, G., G. Giustina, F. Degos, et al. (1997). Morbidity and mortality in compensated cirrhosis type C: a retrospective follow-up study of 384 patients. *Gastroenterology, 112*(2), 463–472.

Ghany, M. G., D. B. Strader, D. L. Thomas, & L. B. Seeff (2009). Diagnosis, management, and treatment of hepatitis C: an update. *Hepatology, 49*(4), 1335–1374.

Hu, K. Q., & M. J. Tong (1999). The long-term outcomes of patients with compensated hepatitis C virus-related cirrhosis and history of parenteral exposure in the United States. *Hepatology, 29*(4), 1311–1316.

John-Baptiste, A., M. Krahn, J. Heathcote, A. Laporte, & G. Tomlinson (2010). The natural history of hepatitis C infection acquired through injection drug use: meta-analysis and meta-regression. *Journal of Hepatology, 53*(2), 245–251.

Lavanchy, D. (2009). The global burden of hepatitis C. *Liver International, 29*(Suppl 1), 74–81.

Liang, T. J., B. Rehermann, L. B. Seeff, P., & J. H. Hoofnagle (2000). Pathogenesis, natural history, treatment, and prevention of hepatitis C. *Annals of Internal Medicine, 132*(4), 296–305.

Poynard, T., P. Bedossa, & P. Opolon (1997). Natural history of liver fibrosis progression in patients with chronic hepatitis C. The OBSVIRC, METAVIR, CLINIVIR, and DOSVIRC groups. *Lancet, 349*(9055), 825–832.

Chapter 8

Extrahepatic Manifestations of Hepatitis C

Suzanne Robertazzi and Anjana A. Pillai

Introduction

Since the identification of the hepatitis C virus (HCV), several associations have been discovered between the virus and a variety of extrahepatic clinical manifestations (Table 8.1). Studies report that up to 40% of patients with chronic hepatitis C infection have at least one extrahepatic manifestation (Meyer & Bodenheimer, 2009; Zignego & Craxi, 2008). Extrahepatic manifestations have been theorized to trigger clinical disease in numerous organ systems, causing renal, vascular, endocrine, rheumatologic, dermatologic, neurologic, and ophthalmologic involvement (Sterling & Bralow, 2006). This review will highlight three extrahepatic manifestations that have well-documented correlations with hepatitis C viremia: mixed cryoglobulinemia, B-cell lymphoma, and porphyria cutanea tarda.

Mixed Cryoglobulinemia

Case: 55-year-old Caucasian woman with genotype 1b hepatitis C was evaluated for a new purpuric rash on her bilateral lower extremities and significant proteinuria. Patient had a recent liver biopsy that showed chronic hepatitis C with grade 3 inflammation and stage 3 fibrosis. Her HCV viral load was 212,785 IU/mL. Her cryoglobulin screen was positive. A renal biopsy revealed "cryoglobulinemic hepatitis C-associated membranoproliferative glomerulonephritis." Patient was started on antiviral therapy with pegylated interferon alpha (PEG IFN-α) 2a and ribavirin (RBV). Her proteinuria and rash resolved after 8 weeks of treatment. Unfortunately, her 12-week viral load did not reflect a two-log drop, and treatment was discontinued. Her vasculitis reappeared several months after treatment discontinuation.

Mixed cryoglobulinemia (MC) is the most common extrahepatic manifestation associated with HCV and is characterized by the deposition of circulating immune complexes in the small vessels of various organs, leading to a systemic vasculitis. Cryoglobulin complexes were first described in the literature in 1966 by Meltzer and Franklin in a group of patients who expressed the triad of purpura, arthralgia, and weakness without an identifiable underlying disease

Table 8.1 **Extrahepatic Manifestations of Chronic Hepatitis C Infection**

- Mixed cryoglobulinemia
- Non-Hodgkin's lymphoma
- Membranoproliferative glomerulonephritis
- Leukocytoclastic vasculitis
- Porphyria cutanea tarda
- Lichen planus
- Thyroid abnormalities
- Diabetes mellitus
- Sicca syndrome
- Autoantibodies
- Peripheral neuropathy
- Neurocognitive dysfunction
- Idiopathic pulmonary fibrosis

process (Meltzer & Franklin, 1966). MC is believed to be an HCV-related lymphoproliferative disorder.

Cryoglobulins are circulating immunoglobulins that precipitate when serum is cooled below core body temperature and resolubilize when warmed. They are classified into three subtypes. Type I is composed of monoclonal immunoglobulins and frequently associated with hematologic malignancies. Type II is composed of polyclonal IgG and monoclonal IgM, and type III is composed of polyclonal IgG and polyclonal IgM (Charles & Dustin, 2009). HCV is primarily seen with type II MC.

MC can involve multiple organ systems, affecting the small and medium-sized vessels of the skin, peripheral nerves, kidneys, and salivary and lacrimal glands (Charles & Dustin, 2009; Zignego & Craxi, 2008). Serum cryoglobulins have been detected in 40% to 60% of patients with HCV (Lunel et al., 1994; Pawlotsky et al., 1994), yet only 10% to 15% of these patients develop symptomatic MC (Saadoun et al., 2007). The reason for this discrepancy remains unknown. In addition, patients with MC have a higher incidence of advanced fibrosis and cirrhosis compared to patients without detectable cryoglobulins (Kayali et al., 2002; Lunel et al., 1994).

Because of its variable presentation, there are no standardized criteria for the diagnosis of MC. Typically, the diagnosis is made when patients present with clinical manifestations in the setting of positive serum cryoglobulins. An elevated rheumatoid factor and reduced C4 counts may also be useful to confirm the diagnosis (Zignego & Craxi, 2008). Some patients may show clinical symptoms of MC without having detectable serum cryoglobulins (Zignego & Graxi, 2008). Improper collection and transport of samples are the most common reasons for a false-negative cryoglobulin screen.

The most common manifestation of HCV-associated MC is palpable purpura of the lower extremities, where venous stasis favors the precipitation of cryoglobulins. This rash is often preceded by paresthesias (Charles & Dustin, 2009; Meyer & Bodenheimer, 2009). Additional symptoms include arthralgias, fatigue, and weakness. Purpuric lesions may progress to large chronic necrotic ulcers. Membranoproliferative glomerulonephritis, the renal manifestation of MC, can occur in up to one third of patients. Findings range from arterial hypertension, isolated proteinuria (usually in the non-nephrotic range), microscopic hematuria, and mild renal insufficiency to progressive renal failure (Charles & Dustin, 2009; Zignego & Craxi, 2008). The presence of renal involvement is a negative prognostic factor in patients with MC. Neurologic involvement can result in painful paresthesias and concomitant weakness leading to a foot or wrist drop (Charles & Dustin, 2009).

The most effective treatment for MC is eradication of the HCV infection. Traditionally, maintenance therapy used to consist of corticosteroids, cytotoxic agents (cyclophosphamide, AZA), and plasmapheresis, with limited success. Current first-line therapy consists of standard courses of PEG IFN and RBV. For patients who do not respond to initial therapy, extending treatment to 48 weeks for genotype 2/3 and 72 weeks for genotype 1/4 should be considered in the setting of symptomatic improvement (Zignego et al., 2007). Symptoms typically resolve when a sustained virologic response (SVR) has been achieved (Viganoi et al., 2011), although there are reports of symptom persistence even after SVR.

Rituximab has also been successfully used in patients with symptomatic MC who are treatment failures or intolerant to PEG IFN and RBV (Pietrogrande et al., 2011). Rituximab is a chimeric monoclonal antibody against the protein CD20, which is primarily found on the surface of B cells. Rituximab is generally safe and well tolerated, although it has been associated with a significant increase in HCV viral load (Pietrogrande et al., 2011; Saadoun et al., 2008).

Short courses of low-dose corticosteroids may be considered to control vasculitic flares in patients who do not respond to first-line treatments. Corticosteroids are not recommended for continuous suppressive therapy given their deleterious side effects, including enhancing HCV replication (Pietrogrande et al., 2011) (Fig. 8.1).

B-Cell Lymphoma

Case: 68-year-old Hispanic woman with genotype 2 hepatitis C and stage 1 fibrosis on biopsy was admitted for abdominal pain and found to have a hypoproliferative anemia. A CT scan of the abdomen and pelvis was noncontributory. She underwent a bone marrow biopsy, which was consistent with a B-cell lymphoproliferative disorder. She also underwent a renal biopsy for acute renal failure with proteinuria and hematuria. Her renal biopsy also confirmed focal kidney involvement by a low-grade B-cell lymphoma. She was started on treatment with PEG IFN-α 2a and RBV. She achieved a rapid virologic response and completed 6 months of treatment. She subsequently achieved a SVR and her

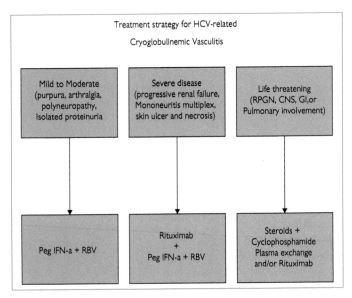

Figure 8.1 Pathogenesis of hepatitis C virus-related lymphoproliferative disorders: an evidence-based hypothesis. (From Figure 1, p. 619, in A. L. Zignego & A. Craxi [2008]. Extrahepatic manifestations of hepatitis C virus infection. *Clinics in Liver Disease, 12*[3], 611–636.)

lymphoma was found to be in remission without any evidence of malignancy on repeat bone marrow biopsy.

HCV, in addition to its hepatotropic properties, has known tropism for peripheral lymphocytes. It has been shown that the HCV envelope protein E2 binds to B lymphocytes via the tetraspanin CD81. This interaction is believed to lower the activation threshold of these cells, leading to chronic antigenic stimulation. This subsequently may lead to polyclonal B-cell expansion, progression to autonomous B-cell proliferation, immune dysregulation, and malignant transformation leading to the development of malignant lymphoma (Medina et al., 2004; Zignego et al., 2007). Another theory is that HCV induces mutagenesis, which leads to prolonged B-cell survival and eventual malignant transformation. Genetic and environmental factors are also believed to play a key role in the formation of B-cell lymphoma. Although the exact mechanism remains unclear, there is an undeniably strong link between HCV and B-cell lymphomas.

HCV viremia has been reported in up to 35% of patients with B-cell lymphoma, and almost 90% of non-Hodgkin's lymphoma (NHL) patients have detectable cryoglobulins (Galossi et al., 2007). MC patients have an estimated 35 times higher risk of NHL compared to the general population (Monti et al., 2005). Approximately 8% to 10% of patients with HCV-associated MC will progress to a high-grade lymphoma (Zignego & Craxi, 2008). Marginal-zone lymphoma appears to be the most frequently encountered low-grade B-cell lymphoma in HCV patients (Viswanatha & Dogan, 2007). Among these there is an especially strong association between HCV and mucosa-associated lymphoid tissue (MALT) lymphoma (Meyer & Bodenheimer, 2009). Additionally, approximately 65% of HCV-related lymphomas have extranodal involvement, particularly in the salivary glands and the liver, compared to only 19% of non-HCV-related lymphomas (Viswanatha & Dogan, 2007).

Antiviral therapy is a reasonable approach to the treatment of patients with low-grade HCV-associated lymphoma. PEG IFN-based treatments have been shown to cause regression of these low-grade lymphomas after viral clearance (Viswanatha & Dogan, 2007). However, this is not the case with intermediate or high-grade lymphomas, where systemic chemotherapy remains the mainstay of treatment and antiviral therapy may be used for maintenance therapy (Gisbert et al., 2005). The use of rituximab as monotherapy or in combination with antiviral therapy and/or chemotherapy is also being studied. Small studies have shown successful use of rituximab monotherapy as first-line therapy for HCV-related indolent B-cell lymphoma (Hainsworth et al., 2002).

Porphyria Cutanea Tarda

Case: 49-year-old Caucasian man with newly diagnosed genotype 2b hepatitis C presented to clinic with a blistering rash on both of his hands. He was initially treated by his primary care physician with cortisone cream, which did not provide any relief. He was referred to a dermatologist, who gave him the diagnosis of porphyria cutanea tarda. His physical exam revealed numerous purple lesions on both his hands. There were no other lesions found on his body. Of note, laboratory values showed a significantly elevated ferritin of 1,508, negative cryoglobulin screen, and a HCV viral load of 413,852 IU/mL. His total plasma porphyrins and 24-hour urine porphyrins were markedly elevated. A liver biopsy showed chronic hepatitis with mild chronic inflammatory activity and stage 1 fibrosis. Iron stain showed 2-3+ iron in both hepatocytes and Kupffer cells. Therapeutic phlebotomy was initiated for his elevated ferritin, with subsequent normalization of his levels and improvement of his skin lesions. Antiviral therapy with PEG IFN-α 2a and RBV was started shortly afterwards. He achieved a complete early virologic response and subsequently attained a SVR. He did not have any further recurrence of his skin lesions.

Porphyria cutanea tarda (PCT) is a disorder characterized by reduced activity of uroporphyrinogen decarboxylase, an enzyme in the heme biosynthetic pathway. It is the most common of the porphyrias. It is associated with skin fragility, bullae formation, hypertrichosis of light-exposed areas, hyperpigmentation, sclerodermoid changes, dystrophic calcifications with ulcerations, scarring, alopecia, and onycholysis (Dienhart & Sterling, 2005; Sterling & Bralow, 2006). These lesions occur due to the photosensitizing effect of porphyrins that accumulate in the skin.

The exact effect of HCV on PCT is unknown but is believed to be related to HCV-induced hepatic iron overload. Development of PCT likely requires a combination of genetic, infectious, and environmental factors. HCV is the most common viral infection associated with PCT. In the United States alone, approximately 56% of patients with PCT have HCV, as opposed to only 2% of the general population (Dienhart & Sterling, 2005; Rebora, 2010).

The diagnosis of PCT is based on increased uro-carboxyl porphyrins and heptacarboxyporphyrins in the urine in addition to elevated liver function tests, ferritin, and serum iron (Rebora, 2010). A 24-urine porphyrin level of more than 2 micromoles suggests extensive liver accumulation of porphyrin. Liver biopsy findings include increased intracellular porphyrins or red fluorescence of biopsy tissue with long-wave ultraviolet light scans (Dienhart & Sterling, 2005).

Physical exam findings include erythema, skin fragility, bullae, erosions, and hypertrichosis. Blisters, vesicles, and milia are seen on the dorsal surface of the extremities, especially the hands and other photo-exposed areas (Rebora, 2010; Sterling & Bralow, 2006).

Treatment consists of lifestyle modifications, including sun avoidance or judicious use of sun block and protective clothing (Sterling & Bralow, 2006). Therapeutic phlebotomy can be used to lower serum ferritin levels, which typically requires twice-weekly treatments for 2 to 3 months. Resolution of blisters is often seen in the first few months; however, reduction in skin fragility may take up to 9 months and normalization of porphyrin concentrations may take over a year (Dienhart & Sterling, 2005). Therapeutic phlebotomy should be considered prior to PEG IFN and RBV treatment. Careful consideration should be made prior to using phlebotomy in conjunction with RBV, as the combination can lead to severe anemia. Currently, there are no standardized trials to determine the appropriate timing between discontinuing phlebotomy and starting antiviral therapy.

Several case reports have shown the resolution of PCT once a SVR has been achieved. Interestingly, there have also been few case reports that document *de novo* occurrence of PCT during PEG IFN and RBV therapy for chronic HCV (Azim et al., 2008).

Conclusion

It is important to consider a multidisciplinary approach to treating patients with extrahepatic manifestations of chronic hepatitis C infection. These coexisting disease entities can add to the complexity of antiviral therapy, and the additional input from rheumatology, dermatology, nephrology, and oncology can help guide treatment and manage added side effects.

There are no current data using HCV protease inhibitors in the above conditions, and as such, recommendations for their use cannot be made at this time. It is anticipated that studies testing the effectiveness of protease inhibitors will be available in the near future.

References

Azim, J., H. McCurdy, & R. Moseley (2008). Porphyria cutanea tarda as a complication of therapy for chronic hepatitis C. *World Journal of Gastroenterology, 14,* 5913–5915.

Charles, E., & L. Dustin (2009). Hepatitis C virus-induced cryoglobulinemia. *International Society of Nephrology, 76,* 818–824.

Dienhart, P., & R. Sterling (2005). Management of hepatitis C virus in patients with porphyria cutanea tarda. *Current Hepatitis Reports 4,* 104–111.

Galossi, A., R. Guarisco, L. Bellis, & C. Puoti (2007). Extrahepatic manifestations of chronic HCV infection. *Journal of Gastrointestinal Liver Disease, 16,* 65–73.

Gisbert, J. P., L. Garcia-Buey, J. M. Pajares, et al. (2005). Systematic review: regression of lymphoproliferative disorders after treatment for hepatitis C infection. *Alimentary Pharmacology & Therapeutics, 21,* 653–662.

Hainsworth, J. D., S. Litchy, H. A. Burris III, et al. (2002). Rituximab as first-line and maintenance therapy for patients with indolent non-Hodgkin's lymphoma. *Journal of Clinical Oncology, 20,* 4261–4267.

Kayali, Z., V. E. Buckwold, B. Zimmerman, & W. N. Schmidt (2002). Hepatitis C, cryoglobulinemia, and cirrhosis: a meta-analysis. *Hepatology, 36*(4), 978–985.

Lunel, F., L. Musset, P. Cacoub, L. Frangeul, P. Cresta, et al. (1994). Cryoglobulinemia in chronic liver diseases: role of hepatitis C virus and liver damage. *Gastroenterology, 106,* 1291–1300.

Medina, J., L. Garc'a-Buey, & R. Moreno-Otero (2004). Hepatitis C virus-related extrahepatic disease—aetiopathogenesis and management. *Alimentary Pharmacology & Therapeutics, 20*(2), 129–141.

Meltzer, M., & E. C. Franklin (1966). Cryoglobulinemia—a study of twenty-nine patients. I. IgG and IgM cryoglobulins and factors affecting cryoprecipitability. *American Journal of Medicine, 40*(6), 828–836.

Meyer, D., & H. Bodenheimer (2009). Extrahepatic manifestations of chronic hepatitis C infection. In: K. Shetty & G. Wu (Eds.), *Clinical gastroenterology: Chronic viral hepatitis* (pp. 135–157). New York: Humana Press.

Monti, G., P. Pioltelli, F. Saccardo, M. Campanini, M. Candela, et al. (2005). Incidence and characteristics of non-Hodgkin lymphomas in a multicenter case file of patients with hepatitis C virus-related symptomatic mixed cryoglobulinemias. *Archives of Internal Medicine, 165*(1), 101–105.

Pawlotsky, J. M., M. Ben Yahia, C. Andre, M. C. Voisin, L. Intrator, et al. (1994). Immunological disorders in C virus chronic active hepatitis: a prospective case-control study. *Hepatology, 19,* 841–848.

Pietrogrande, M., et al. (2011). Recommendations for the management of mixed cryoglobulinemia syndrome in hepatitis C virus-infected patients. *Autoimmunity Reviews, 10,* 444–454.

Rebora, A. (2010). Skin diseases associated with hepatitis C virus: facts and controversies. *Clinics in Dermatology, 28,* 489–496.

Saadoun, D., D. A. Landau, L. H. Calabrese, & P. P. Cacoub (2007). Hepatitis C-associated mixed cryoglobulinaemia: a crossroad between autoimmunity and lymphoproliferation. *Rheumatology, 46,* 1234–1242.

Saadoun, D., A. Delluc, J. Piette, & P. Cacoub (2008). Treatment of hepatitis c-associated mixed cryoglobulinemia vasculitis. *Current Opinion in Rheumatology, 20,* 23–28.

Sterling, R., & P. Bralow (2006). Extrahepatic manifestations of hepatitis C virus. *Current Gastroenterology Reports, 8,* 53–59.

Viganoi, A., et al. (2011). The association of cryoglobulinaemia with sustained virological response in patients with chronic hepatitis C. *Journal of Viral Hepatitis,18,* e91–e98.

Viswanatha, D., & A. Dogan (2007). Hepatitis C virus and lymphoma. *Journal of Clinical Pathology, 60,* 1378–1383.

Zignego, A., C. Giannini, & C. Ferri (2007). Hepatitis C virus-related lymphoproliferative disorders: an overview. *World Journal of Gastroenterology, 13*(17), 2467–2478.

Zignego, A. L., & Crax`, A. (2008). Extrahepatic manifestations of hepatitis C virus infection. *Clinics in Liver Disease, 12*(3), 611–636.

Chapter 9

Hepatitis C in Liver Transplantation

Leila Kia, Kristina A. Matkowskyj, and Josh Levitsky

Introduction

Hepatitis C infection is the leading indication worldwide for orthotopic liver transplantation (OLT). All HCV-infected liver transplant recipients invariably develop recurrence, ranging from histologic evidence of mild inflammation to fibrosing cholestatic hepatitis (FCH), an accelerated recurrence of cirrhosis associated with extremely poor outcomes (Satapathy et al., 2011). Risk factors for recurrence, optimal treatment, the role of prophylaxis, and indications for retransplantation are matters of ongoing research and debate.

Epidemiology and Risk Factors for Recurrence

The majority of OLT recipients develop histologic evidence of recurrence within 5 years of OLT. Within this group, 10% to 25% develop evidence of cirrhosis in the transplanted liver, while an even smaller number develop FCH. This has led to the standard practice of performing routine liver biopsies 1 to 2 years following OLT to monitor the degree of recurrence post-transplantation. Once HCV cirrhosis recurs, 40% of patients decompensate within 1 year, resulting in 1- and 4-year patient survival rates of 66% and 33% respectively, highlighting the importance of close post-transplant monitoring.

Risk factors for accelerated HCV recurrence are shown in Table 9.1 (Levitsky & Doucette, 2009).

The best-identified risk factors for HCV recurrence relate to acute rejection therapy and the use of intravenous corticosteroids and lymphodepleting antibodies in the perioperative period. Cytomegalovirus (CMV) infection and ischemia–reperfusion injury also have a clear association with rapid recurrence.

Risk factors associated with the donor are also significant in predicting HCV recurrence. Due to the high demand for donor livers, various strategies have been implemented to expand the donor pool, including the use of marginal or expanded donor livers for transplantation. This includes using donors after cardiac death (DCD), donors greater than 60 years of age, and HCV-infected donors. The impact on outcomes and recurrence in post-OLT HCV patients has been variable. Studies have shown that recipients of older donor livers

Table 9.1 Risk Factors for Accelerated HCV Recurrence		
Definite	**Controversial**	**Not Clearly Associated**
Acute rejection therapy:	Corticosteroid therapy	Induction therapy
Intravenous steroids	Use vs. complete	IL-2 antibody
Lymphodepleting	avoidance	Lymphodepleting antibody
antibody	Rapid vs. slow tapering	HCV+ donor
Donor age	Viral load (>1 × 10^6	Live donor
Recipient age	copies/mL at transplant)	Maintenance
Cytomegalovirus	Genotype 1b	immunosuppression
infection	Donor after cardiac death	
Ischemia–reperfusion	HLA mismatch	
injury		
Diabetes mellitus		

(>60 years) and DCD livers (particularly from DCD donors that are older) have worse outcomes, including immediate perioperative complications and recurrent HCV-related cirrhosis/decompensation (Alonso et al., 2005; Yagci et al., 2008). In DCD donors, HCV recurrence has been shown to be more rapid, but graft failure and patient survival rates do not appear to be affected. Data from the Organ Procurement and Transplant Network (OPTN) show that HCV-positive DCD recipients have 1- and 3-year patient survival rates of 84% and 75%, while HCV-negative DCD recipients have rates of 84% and 76% respectively, suggesting no difference. The data for older donors are not as favorable. Both recurrence and patient survival are affected negatively by donor age of more than 60 years. The mechanism by which older age is associated with poor outcomes is not well established, but is likely multifactorial. Older-donor livers have a lower tolerance for preservation and a greater susceptibility to cold ischemia. Furthermore, age-related immune changes, such as liver steatosis, iron content, preexisting fibrosis, and changes in telomeres/ senescence may play a role in accelerating recurrence (Berenguer, 2008). The current consensus recommendation is that donors over 60 years of age should not be used for HCV-positive recipients. However, DCD donors younger than 60 years of age (and particularly <40) are still being transplanted in this subset of patients and appear to have acceptable outcomes. Finally, the HCV status of the donor has also been evaluated in predicting recurrence. Superinfection with the donor HCV strain has been described in the recipient and does not appear to affect survival or recurrence of HCV. Progression of HCV disease is similar to that in patients receiving uninfected grafts. Interestingly, recipients who retain their strain appear to have more severe liver disease (Berenguer, 2008; Samuel et al., 2006). Of note, transplanting genotype 1 HCV-positive donors into non-genotype 1 recipients is not recommended.

Other factors predisposing to increased risk that have no conclusive evidence include female gender, donor hypernatremia, prolonged hospitalization, African-American race, and pressor requirement perioperatively (Feng et al., 2006).

Diagnosis

Monitoring of liver function tests (LFT) following OLT is done routinely, but abnormalities are common and do not differentiate between HCV recurrence and other etiologies of LFT abnormalities, particularly allograft rejection. The gold standard for diagnosing recurrence versus rejection is liver biopsy, which is done routinely in most transplant centers 1 to 2 years following OLT. However, despite being the gold standard, histologic evaluation of the allograft is often not specific enough to differentiate between recurrence and early graft dysfunction and may inaccurately state the degree of fibrosis (Skripenova et al., 2007).

To evaluate for acute rejection, pathologists rely on the Banff criteria, looking for the presence of a mixed portal inflammatory infiltrate composed of lymphocytes, eosinophils, and neutrophils, along with ductilitis and endothelialitis with minimal hepatocyte damage (Fig. 9.1). In chronic rejection, there is loss of intrahepatic/interlobular bile ducts, subintimal fibrosis, and foam cell changes in large- and medium-caliber hilar hepatic arteries and portal veins (Fig. 9.2). Due to technical limitations, the diagnostic vascular changes are rarely present in needle biopsy specimens.

Histologic features of HCV recurrence in the liver allograft are similar to those in a nontransplanted liver and can present as early, established, or progressive changes. In the early phase, there is mild, nonspecific portal inflammation. An established infection presents as acute hepatitis approximately 2 to 4 months post-transplantation. The histologic findings include lobular hepatocyte disarray, ballooning change, and Mallory bodies (Fig. 9.3). With progressive

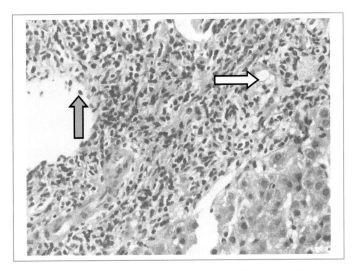

Figure 9.1 Acute cellular rejection. Portal tract with mixed inflammatory infiltrate composed of lymphocytes, neutrophils and eosinophils. There is damage to the bile ducts (white arrow) and undermining/sloughing of the venous endothelium (blue arrow).

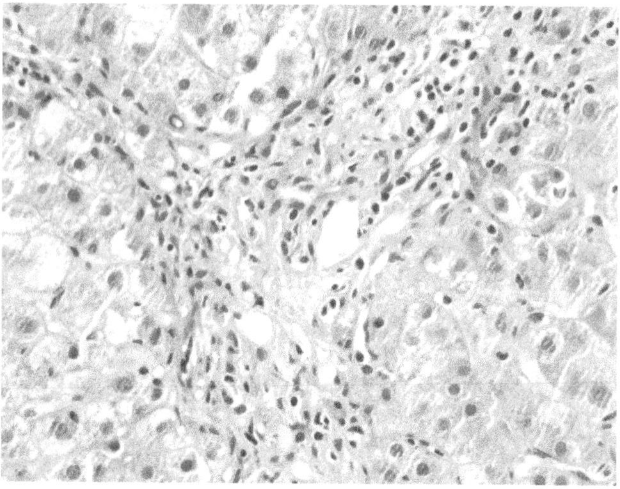

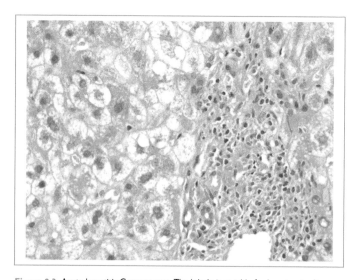

Figure 9.2 Chronic ductopenic rejection. This portal tract demonstrates the loss of an intrahepatic/interlobular bile duct with minimal portal inflammation.

Figure 9.3 Acute hepatitis C recurrence. The lobule is notable for hepatocyte disarray, ballooning change, and the presence of Mallory bodies. Within the portal tract, there is minimal inflammation composed of lymphocytes and plasma cells. No evidence of acute rejection is seen.

infection, there is a predominantly portal infiltrate composed of lymphocytes often with lymphoid follicle formation, the presence of occasional plasma cells and/or eosinophils, and focal mild macrovesicular fatty change with minimal acidophil bodies (Fig. 9.4). When compared to the nontransplanted patient, the course of HCV is often more aggressive with recurrence in the allograft as demonstrated by more severe inflammatory activity and rapid progression to

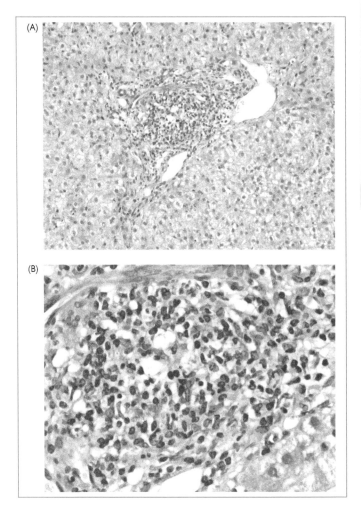

Figure 9.4 Recurrent hepatitis C. (A) Predominantly portal inflammatory infiltrate with minimal lobular activity. (B) Lymphoid follicle formation composed of lymphocytes with an occasional plasma cell.

fibrosis, with a 5-year risk of cirrhosis ranging from 8% to 28%. Certain features in early post-transplant biopsies may suggest a more rapid progression to fibrosis and include severity of necroinflammatory activity, presence and severity of macrovesicular steatosis in day 1 to 28 biopsies, and presence of prominent hepatocyte ballooning and cholestasis (Samuel et al., 2006).

Because some post-transplant biopsies may have histologic patterns that overlap between the findings present in recurrence as well as rejection, other supportive tests are used in conjunction with the biopsy findings to aid in the diagnosis of HCV recurrence. These include measurement of the hepatic venous pressure gradient (HVPG) and measurement of liver stiffness. An elevated HVPG (>10 mmHg) suggests development of portal hypertension and has been shown to predict progression to more advanced disease (Blasco et al., 2006; Kalambokis et al., 2009). Liver stiffness, as measured by transient elastography, offers a noninvasive measure of fibrosis and has a higher sensitivity and positive predictive value for advanced fibrosis compared to other clinical markers (Carrion et al., 2006). Overall, no sole test is sufficient to provide an accurate assessment of disease progression; however, the use of combined modalities can allow for more accurate predictions. Histologic evidence of recurrence, as described above, and/or the degree of liver stiffness as measured by elastography, along with evidence of portal hypertension as measured by the HVPG, are indicative of disease progression and HCV recurrence. These modalities and findings may be useful in providing prognostic information and aid in the decision-making process for treatment purposes.

Treatment

Pretransplant

A viral load greater than 1×10^6 copies/mL at transplant is likely associated with a higher risk of rapid HCV recurrence. Clearance of HCV viremia resulting in a sustained virologic response (SVR) prior to OLT may delay the need for OLT and reduce the risk of recurrence. With the standard therapy of pegylated interferon (PEG-IFN) and ribavirin (RBV), approximately 42% to 52% of genotype 1 patients and 76% to 84% of genotype 2/3 patients achieve SVR (Fried et al., 2002). However, with the recent introduction of the protease inhibitors boceprevir and telaprevir, triple therapy for genotype 1 HCV patients will likely become standard of care, given the much higher rates of SVR seen with combination therapy (approximately 75%) (Jacobson et al., 2011; Poordad et al., 2011). This will likely reduce the number of patients requiring OLT while increasing the number of patients who achieve SVR prior to undergoing OLT, thus helping reduce the risk of rapid HCV recurrence.

Post-transplant

Treatment of recurrence of HCV in post-transplant patients has traditionally been with IFN or PEG-IFN + RBV, but data suggest that it is successful in only approximately 20% to 30% of patients and is associated with a high rate of discontinuation secondary to intolerance (Wang et al., 2006). A major limiting factor in achieving SVR in post-transplant patients is the presence of renal insufficiency, which limits the target RBV doses needed to achieve SVR. No studies as of yet have looked at the use of protease inhibitors in post-transplant treatment, but these will likely be forthcoming with the recent introduction of these novel agents.

Prophylaxis

In the broadest sense, prophylaxis involves reducing the risk factors known to increase the risk of rapid HCV recurrence, including acute rejection, use of extended-criteria or older donors, and CMV infection, as discussed above. Another approach to prophylaxis/prevention of HCV recurrence is the consideration of prophylactic treatment with PEG-IFN and RBV post-transplantation. Multiple studies have been carried out to evaluate this approach, all of which have shown disappointing results. A recent large multicenter randomized controlled trial (PHOENIX) found no significant difference in the rate of HCV recurrence at 120 weeks in patients who had undergone prophylactic treatment with PEG-IFN and RBV compared to those who had undergone observation only (Bzowei et al., 2011). Interestingly, there was also no difference in the rates of acute rejection between the two groups, which is often a concern when treating post-transplant patients with interferon. The current recommendations are not to treat HCV recipients prophylactically post-OLT. With the introduction of the directly acting antivirals boceprevir and telaprevir, it will be interesting to see if further studies using triple therapy will show similar results.

Retransplantation

The decision to relist a patient with recurrent HCV cirrhosis post-OLT is done on a case-by-case basis and remains a controversial issue among transplant centers. Observational studies have shown that patients with rapid recurrence who are retransplanted have poor outcomes and nearly universally recur quickly after retransplantation. In an era of continued organ shortage, the decision to relist a patient with HCV recurrence is a difficult one. Studies have tried to identify patients who may benefit from retransplantation, comparing outcomes to retransplantation for non-HCV patients. A recent study comparing HCV retransplants versus non-HCV retransplants (excluding primary nonfunction) showed no difference in survival between the two groups. The same study looked at predictive factors of poor outcomes and found significant trends in elevated bilirubin, AST, and white cell counts on day of transplant, which correlated with shorter survival (Bahra et al., 2007). At this time, transplant centers continue to retransplant patients with rapid recurrence on a case-by-case basis.

Fibrosing Cholestatic Hepatitis

FCH is a rare but severe form of recurrent HCV that portends a grim prognosis for the recipient. It is characterized by severe cholestatic injury and rapidly progressive liver dysfunction. It is seen in approximately 5% to 10% of post-OLT HCV-positive recipients. Most cases are fatal despite attempts at treatment and changes in immunosuppression. The entity was first identified in the 1990s in recipients with hepatitis B but has since been well documented in HCV recipients. The first histologic account in the literature described a pattern of "extensive dense portal fibrosis with immature fibrous bands extending into sinusoidal spaces, ductal proliferation and hypercellularity, marked canalicular and cellular cholestasis, and moderate mononuclear inflammation" (Davies et al., 1991) (Fig. 9.5). This description is not particularly specific to FCH. Today, distinguishing FCH from other forms of hepatitis remains a challenge and cannot rely solely on histologic interpretation, but rather combines clinical, biochemical, and serologic profiles.

One important challenge when reviewing post-OLT complications is to distinguish FCH from acute cellular rejection. Some histologic clues can aid in differentiating the two. In FCH, the earliest changes are typically lobular without significant changes in the portal area, which are more typical in acute cellular rejection, including endothelialitis, ductilitis, and a mixed portal-inflammatory infiltrate. The initial changes in FCH include centrilobular (zone 3) hepatocyte ballooning degeneration with mild inflammatory activity. The degree of cholestasis can vary at this stage. As the disease progresses, portal changes become more prominent, and bile ductular proliferation and portal expansion due to the mixed inflammatory infiltrate occurs. The degree of fibrosis then progresses from pericellular and perisinusoidal to bridging fibrosis, and in some cases to cirrhosis. Chronic graft rejection can also lead to cholestasis and may be hard to distinguish from FCH. In the former, foam cell changes and a lack of intrahepatic/interlobular bile ducts are prominent (see Fig. 9.1), which are not typical of FCH. The timing of the changes may also help distinguish between acute rejection, chronic rejection, and FCH, although FCH can occur across all timelines (Narang et al., 2010). New tools, such as assessment of biopsies for hepatic stellate activation (via immunostaining), may also help distinguish cases of FCH (Dixon & Crawford, 2007). Despite the difficulty in distinguishing between FCH and forms of rejection, it is imperative to distinguish FCH from acute cellular rejection, as escalation of immunosuppression can be devastating for a patient with FCH.

Unfortunately, there are no clearly established risk factors for developing FCH, so it is impossible to predict who will develop this complication. Patients who have undergone combined liver/kidney transplants have been noted to have a higher rate of FCH at some centers, though the reason for this is unclear. Genotype, type of immunosuppression, and HCV viral load have also been suggested as risk factors, but the data on these have been equivocal. The pathogenesis for FCH is poorly understood, but a proposed mechanism involves hepatocyte repopulation and regeneration after liver transplantation (Honda et al., 2000). Injury of hepatocytes is thought to be from a direct cytopathic effect of HCV, wherein there is a relative absence of inflammation, a high serum viral load, and many HCV virions in the hepatocytes. After transplantation, within hours of graft reperfusion, the thought is that there is a repopulation of the viral load to pretransplant levels, which leads to the rapid cytopathic effect. Interestingly, studies have shown that patients with mild recurrent HCV

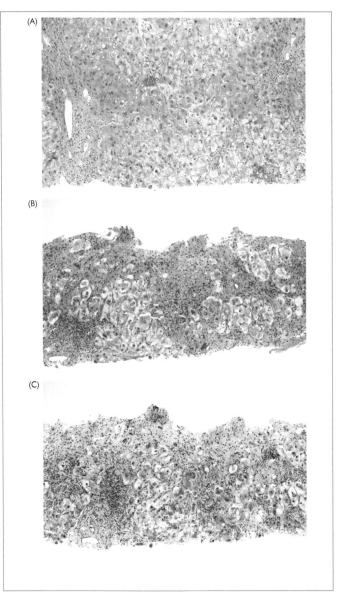

Figure 9.5 Fibrosing cholestatic hepatitis. (A) Biopsy 15 months post-transplant demonstrates mild portal inflammation, diffuse ballooning change, and mild cholestasis. (B) Biopsy 5 months later (20 months post-transplant) reveals cirrhosis. Confirmation of cirrhosis using Masson's trichrome stain to highlight fibrosis and demonstrated by the blue staining (C).

have more genetic diversification in their genomic RNA viral sequences than patients who develop FCH, suggesting that homogeneity in the viral sequences post-OLT may predispose to FCH.

Outcomes for patients with FCH have been nearly universally grim. Recent studies have suggested that immediate initiation of anti-HCV therapy with PEG-IFN and RBV with conversion from tacrolimus to cyclosporine-based immuno-suppression may have benefits in sustained improvement in hepatic function and survival (Cimsit et al., 2011). Cyclosporine may have antiviral properties and inhibit HCV replication, which may explain the theoretical advantage. No effective treatment has been elucidated to date. Finally, the decision to retransplant these patients is controversial, as they often develop rapid recurrence and FCH following retransplantation.

Conclusion

Hepatitis C recurrence is universal in patients undergoing OLT, and a significant number develop cirrhosis and complications within 5 years of retransplantation. Treatment with PEG-INF and RBV in post-OLT recipients has low success rates, and currently prophylactic treatment has no role in preventing recurrences. FCH is a rare complication and has grim outcomes, with implications in prognosticating graft and patient survival. Retreatment and retransplantation remain the mainstays of management of recurrent HCV cirrhosis. Reduction in risk factors known to accelerate recurrence is also critical in the perioperative period. It will be interesting to see how the introduction of the directly acting antivirals will affect OLT rates for HCV-positive patients. Future studies will also likely evaluate post-transplant prophylaxis and treatment with triple therapy, which may offer better alternatives. Until then, close surveillance and monitoring are critical and individualized decisions need to be made regarding timing of treatment pretransplant, and decisions to treat and retransplant post-OLT.

References

Alonso, O., C. Loinaz, E. Moreno, et al. (2005). Advanced donor age increases the risk of severe recurrent hepatitis C after liver transplantation. *Transplant International, 18,* 902.

Bahra, M., U. P. Neumann, D. Jacob, et al. (2007). Outcome after liver re-transplantation in patients with recurrent chronic hepatitis C. *Transplant International, 20,* 771–778.

Berenguer, M. (2008). Risk of extended criteria donors in hepatitis C virus-positive recipients. *Liver Transplantation, 14,* S45–S50.

Blasco, A., X. Forns, J. A. Carrion, et al. (2006). Hepatic venous pressure gradient identifies patients at risk of severe hepatitis C recurrence after transplantation. *Hepatology, 43,* 492–499.

Bzowej, N., D. R. Nelson, & N. A. Terrault (2011). PHOENIX: A randomized controlled trial of peginterferon alfa-2a plus ribavirin as a prophylactic treatment after liver transplantation for hepatitis C virus. *Liver Transplantation, 17,* 528–538.

Carrion, J. A., M. Navasa, J. Bosch, et al. (2006). Transient elastography for diagnosis of advanced fibrosis and portal hypertension in patients with hepatitis C recurrence after liver transplantation. *Liver Transplantation, 12*, 1791–1798.

Cimsit, B., D. Assis, & C. Caldwell (2011). Successful treatment of fibrosing cholestatic hepatitis after liver transplantation. *Transplantation Proceedings, 43*, 905–908.

Davies, S. E., B. C. Portmann, J. G. O'Grady, et al. (1991). Hepatic histological findings after transplantation for chronic hepatitis B infection, including a unique pattern of fibrosing cholestatic hepatitis. *Hepatology, 13*, 150–157.

Dixon, L. R., & J. M. Crawford (2007). Early histologic changes in fibrosing cholestatic hepatitis C. *Liver Transplantation, 13*, 219–226.

Feng, S., N. P. Goodrich, & J. L. Bragg-Gresham (2006). Characteristics associated with liver graft failure: the concept of the donor risk index. *American Journal of Transplantation, 6*, 783–790.

Fried, M. W., M. L. Shiffman, K. R. Reddy, et al. (2002). Peginterferon alfa-2a plus ribavirin for chronic hepatitis C infection. *New England Journal of Medicine, 34*, 975–982.

Honda, M., S. Kaneko, E. Matsushita, et al. (2000). Cell cycle regulation of HCV internal ribosomal entry site direceted translation. *Gastroenterology, 118*, 152–162.

Jacobson, I. M., J. G. McHutchinson, G. Dusheiko, et al. (2011). Telaprevir for previously untreated chronic hepatitis C virus infection. *New England Journal of Medicine, 364*(25), 2405–2416.

Kalambokis, G., P. Manousou, D. Samonakis, et al. (2009). Clinical outcome of HCV-related graft cirrhosis and prognostic value of hepatic venous pressure gradient. *Transplant International, 22*, 172–181.

Levitsky, J., & K. Doucette (2009). Viral hepatitis in solid organ transplant recipients. *American Journal of Transplantation, 9*(4), S116–S130.

Narang, T. K., W. Ahrens, & M. W. Russo (2010). Post-liver transplant cholestatic hepatitis C: A systematic review of clinical and pathological findings and application of consensus criteria. *Liver Transplantation, 16*, 1228–1235.

Poordad, F., J. McCone, B. R. Bacon, et al. (2011). Boceprevir for untreated chronic HCV genotype 1 infection. *New England Journal of Medicine, 364*(13), 1195–1206.

Samuel, D., X. Forns, M. Berenguer, et al. (2006). Report of the monothematic EASL conference on liver transplantation for viral hepatitis (Paris, France, January 12–14, 2006). *Journal of Hepatology, 45*, 127–143.

Satapathy, S. K., S. Sclair, M. I. Fiel, et al. (2011). Clinical characterization of patients developing histologically-proven fibrosing cholestatic hepatitis C post-liver transplantation. *Hepatology Research, 41*(4), 328–339.

Skripenova, S., T. D. Trainer, E. L. Krawitt, et al. (2007). Variability of grade and stage in simultaneous paired liver biopsies in patients with hepatitis C. *Journal of Clinical Pathology, 60*, 321–324.

Wang, C. S., H. H. Ko, E. M. Yoshida, et al. (2006). Interferon-based combination anti-viral therapy for hepatitis C virus after liver transplantation: a review and quantitative analysis. *American Journal of Transplantation, 6*, 1586–1599.

Yagci, G., S. J. Fernandez, S. J. Knechtle, et al. (2008). The impact of donor variables on the outcomes of orthotopic liver transplantation for hepatitis C. *Transplantation Proceedings, 40*, 219–223.

Chapter 10

Treatment of Hepatitis C

Lesley Dawravoo and Stanley Martin Cohen

Introduction

Hepatitis C (HCV) is a leading cause of liver disease and is a significant burden on the healthcare system (Aronsohn & Reau, 2009). In the United States alone, it is estimated that nearly 3.2 million people are infected with HCV, and it is the leading indication for liver transplant in this country (Armstrong et al., 2006). HCV is seen in approximately 1.6% of the general population, although there is a much higher prevalence in certain subgroups. According to Finnelli and colleagues, 57% of intravenous drug users, 13% of those infected with HIV, and 8% of those on hemodialysis were anti-HCV positive (Finelli et al., 2005). The majority of HCV cases are contracted through injection drug use (60%), although other routes of transmission, including sexual (15%) and through transfusions (10%), are well described (Fig. 10.1) (CDC, 2001).

To date, six major genotypes have been identified. Genotype 1 is the most common in the United States, affecting more than 70% of patients (Kim & Saab, 2005). Genotypes 2 and 3 are less common in the United States and more often seen in Italy, North Africa, Spain, and Northern Europe. Less common genotypes, genotypes 4, 5, and 6, are found in the Middle East, South Africa, and Southeast Asia, respectively (Lauer & Walker, 2001).

Of people who contract HCV, 75% to 85% will go on to develop a chronic infection (Aronsohn & Reau, 2009). Of this group, 20% will progress to cirrhosis, and 20% of cirrhotics will eventually develop hepatocellular carcinoma (HCC). Treatment for HCV is important in order to eradicate the virus, which may prevent, or at least slow, disease progression and the development of associated complications. This chapter will focus on the use of pegylated interferon (PEG-IFN) and ribavirin (RBV). The recently approved direct-acting antiviral HCV therapies will be discussed in a subsequent chapter.

Candidates for HCV Therapy

According to the 2002 NIH Consensus statement, "All patients with chronic hepatitis C are potential candidates for therapy" (NIH, 2002). Ultimately, one wants to achieve a sustained viral response (SVR), which is defined as a negative HCV ribonucleic acid (RNA) level as measured by highly sensitive polymerase chain reaction (PCR) 24 weeks after treatment cessation. Studies have

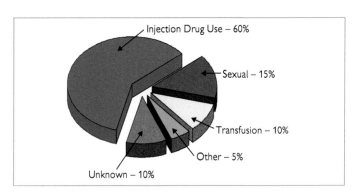

Figure 10.1 Sources of infection in patients with hepatitis C

shown that achieving an SVR leads to improvement in liver histology, slows progression of disease, and decreases the complications of chronic HCV infection (Lindsay, 2002). A recent VA study showed that SVR was associated with a 30% to 49% reduction in all-cause mortality in patients with HCV (Backus et al., 2011). Once an SVR is attained, patients are considered to have a "virologic cure," as rates of SVR have been shown to be durable in 99% to 100% of patients at up to 7 years of follow-up (Fig. 10.2) (Swain et al., 2010).

Certain criteria should be kept in mind when choosing the ideal candidate for treatment. Patients should have a detectable HCV RNA viral load and should have at least moderate inflammation and some fibrosis seen on liver biopsy (Ghany et al., 2009). Other laboratory parameters, including hemoglobin, neutrophil count, and creatinine, should be at acceptable levels, as treatment-related toxicities can affect these values (see below). Cirrhotic patients can be treated but should have compensated liver disease with no evidence of encephalopathy, ascites, or grossly abnormal lab indices (total bilirubin, INR, albumin, and platelets). Due to significant adverse events that can occur with HCV therapy, patients' comorbidities, including hypertension, diabetes mellitus, and coronary artery disease, should be under control. Lastly, the patient needs to be willing to be treated and to adhere to treatment requirements.

Patients in whom treatment is being considered should have no "absolute" contraindications to therapy (Table 10.1) (Heathcote & Main, 2005). There are several "relative" contraindications that also need to be kept in mind. Due to the potential adverse effects of the medicines, treatment may be difficult in those with neutropenia (PMN <750 mm^3), thrombocytopenia (platelets <75,000/mm^3), or anemia (hemoglobin <10 g/dL). Patients with no fibrosis on biopsy may not need therapy. Patients with severe autoimmune disease could see significant flares due to hepatitis C treatment medications. Other relative contraindications include patients actively using alcohol or illicit drugs, those co-infected with HIV, post-transplant patients, or those who have failed previous HCV treatment. Several of these select populations will be discussed in further detail later in the chapter (see "Special Populations" below).

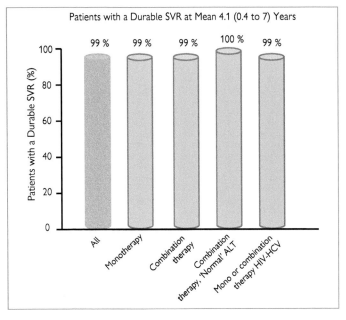

Figure 10.2 Durability of SVR

Table 10.1 Contraindications to Therapy
• Severe/uncontrolled depression
• History of immune-mediated disease
• Untreated thyroid disease
• Age <2 years
• Pregnancy, contemplating pregnancy, unwilling to comply with contraception (even in males)
• Untreated thyroid disease
• Severe uncontrolled comorbidities (diabetes mellitus, coronary artery disease, chronic obstructive pulmonary disease, heart failure, hypertension)
• Known hypersensitivity to the medications

Predictors of Response to HCV Therapy

Several predictors of response need to be considered when treating HCV. The clinician must weigh the risks and benefits of treatment and present all options to the patient. Table 10.2 shows the generally accepted predictors of response, the single most important being viral genotype. On a treatment regimen of

Table 10.2 Predictors of Virologic Response	
Viral Factors	**Host Factors**
• Genotype	• Age
• Viral load	• Race
	• Gender
	• Co-infection (HIV, HBV)
	• Degree of hepatic inflammation or cirrhosis
	• Weight
	• Renal disease
	• Hyperinsulinemia

PEG-IFN and RBV, patients with genotypes 2 and 3 have response rates near 80%, whereas response rates in patients with genotype 1 are in the 40% range (Kim & Saab, 2005). Lower viral loads (HCV RNA <600,000 IU/mL) have been shown to correlate with a higher treatment response rate (Hadzivannis et al., 2004). Patients with pretreatment ALT levels at least three times the upper limit of normal have better response rates. Lower response rates are expected in those with more advanced liver disease or cirrhosis; hence, a liver biopsy prior to therapy can be helpful to guide pretreatment decisions. Ethnicity can also help predict response, as Caucasians have higher response rates than African Americans (see "Special Populations" below). Other factors classically related to a worse response rate include metabolic syndrome and insulin resistance, male patients, and age over 40 years.

A polymorphism has been discovered on chromosome 19 that also predicts SVR rates (Ge et al., 2009; Thomas et al., 2009). This IL28B gene encodes for interferon-lambda 3. Two subtypes, the C allele and the T allele, have been described. Patients with the CC phenotype have been shown to have higher rates of SVR than patients with either CT or TT phenotypes. The exact clinical utility of this test remains unclear.

Pretreatment Testing

As noted above, the level of activity and fibrosis on a liver biopsy may help identify patients who would benefit from HCV therapy as well as predict response to therapy. In addition, the biopsy can rule out concomitant liver disease. Because treatment has complications and the response to therapy is less than 50% in patients with genotype 1, a biopsy may help one decide who *not* to treat. For this reason, a pretreatment liver biopsy is recommended in patients with genotype 1 HCV. However, in patients with genotypes 2 and 3, where response rates are much higher, a biopsy is usually not necessary prior to starting treatment.

Once a patient is deemed an acceptable candidate for therapy, several lab studies should be obtained prior to initiating treatment. All patients should have a CBC, electrolytes, liver function tests, ANA, TSH, and HIV checked. It is also important to have a baseline HCV RNA viral load as well as a genotype.

Because RBV is a known teratogen, female patients should have a pregnancy test. Patients should also have a baseline ophthalmology exam, as IFN can be associated with ophthalmologic adverse events. Testing for hepatitis A and B should be done to rule out co-infection and assess for the need to vaccinate. A thorough neuropsychiatric assessment should be performed. Some experts would also check a baseline ultrasound.

IFN and RBV for the Treatment of HCV

IFNs are proteins with antiviral activity. The alfa-IFNs are the subclass used as treatment of hepatitis C. The actual mechanism of action is not entirely clear, but it is known that alfa-IFNs are able to modulate the cellular immune system and initiate a cytokine cascade. Alfa-IFNs act on specific genes to establish an antiviral state in the cell. They also possess anti-inflammatory properties. The exact mechanism of action of RBV is also not entirely clear. It is known to work as a guanosine nucleoside analog to inhibit viral replication. It is effective against HCV and has activity against other RNA viruses as well.

In its infancy, HCV treatment consisted of monotherapy with standard IFN given three times weekly by subcutaneous injections. SVR rates for 24 weeks of therapy were 6% and improved to only 13% when treatment was extended to 48 weeks (Fig. 10.3) (McHutchison & Poynard, 1999). In the late 1990s, RBV was added to the IFN regimen and SVR rates improved to 31% and 38% at 24 and 48 weeks, respectively. As shown in Figure 10.4, genotype was an important factor in treatment response rates as well as determining length of therapy. In patients with genotype 1, SVR rates improved from 17% to 29% when treatment was extended from 6 months to 12 months, whereas in patients with genotype 2 and 3, SVR rates remained at 65% to 66% with either length of therapy.

One of the theoretical limitations of standard IFN therapy is the fluctuating drug levels due to the short half-life of the medication. In addition to

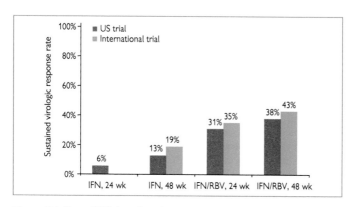

Figure 10.3 Rates of SVR throughout the history of IFN and RBV

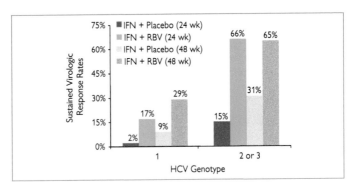

Figure 10.4 Effect of genotype on SVR

Table 10.3 Weight-Based Dosing of Ribavirin	
Genotype 1, 4	**Genotype 2, 3**
• PEG-IFN alfa 2a	• PEG-IFN alfa 2a and 2b
• ≤75 kg = 1,000 mg	• 800 mg daily in divided doses regardless of weight
• >75 kg = 1,200 mg	
• PEG-IFN alfa 2b	
• <65 kg = 800 mg	
• 65–85 kg = 1,000 mg	
• 85–105 kg = 1,200 mg	
• >105 kg = 1,400 mg	

creating peaks and troughs of drug levels, which might have influenced treatment response rates, this medication required multiple injections weekly. A better IFN that would provide constant levels and require fewer injections was then sought. With this concept in mind, PEG-IFN was developed. Pegylation added ethylene glycol to the interferon molecule, which increased the half-life, allowing for once-weekly dosing.

There are currently two FDA-approved forms of PEG-IFN that are used in combination with ribavirin: PEG-IFN alfa-2a (Pegasys), a 40-kD branched polyethylene glycol moiety, and PEG-IFN alfa-2b (Peg-Intron), a 12-kD linear polyethylene glycol moiety. Both are given once weekly as a subcutaneous injection. In all genotypes, PEG-IFN alfa-2a is dosed at 180 µg/week, whereas PEG-IFN alfa-2b is dosed based on weight (1.5 µg/kg/week). RBV also uses weight-based dosing, which differs according to which genotype is being treated and which PEG-IFN product is being used (Table 10.3). The standard course of therapy is 48 weeks for genotype 1 patients and 24 weeks for patients with genotypes 2 and 3.

Using combined PEG-IFN + RBV treatment, overall SVR rates improved to 54% to 56% (Fig. 10.5) (Fried et al., 2002; Manns et al., 2001). Again, genotype

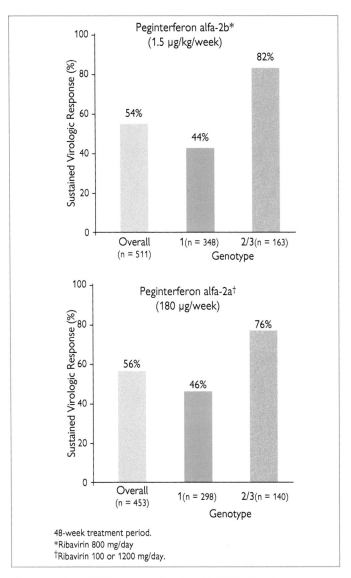

Figure 10.5 Rates of SVR by genotype from the original PEG-IFN registration trial

was noted to be an important factor in SVR rates. SVR rates were 44% to 46% in genotype 1 patients and 76% to 82% in those with genotype 2 or 3. Trials comparing combination therapy with RBV and either PEG-IFN alfa-2a or alfa-2b have shown that rates of SVR are similar between the two PEG-IFNs (Aronsohn & Reau, 2009).

Side Effects of Therapy

There are many side effects associated with the HCV treatment medications (Table 10.4). These adverse events are the most common reason for therapy discontinuation. As shown in the Manns study outlined in Table 10.5, treatment was discontinued in up to 14% of patients and dose reductions were made in up to 42% because of side effects (Manns et al., 2001).

Psychiatric side effects are seen in over one third of patients and may be the most important adverse events, as they are the leading cause of non-adherence to therapy (Fried et al., 2002; Manns et al., 2001). Symptoms may include

Table 10.4 Side Effects of IFN and RBV

- Flu-like Symptoms
  - Headache
  - Fatigue
  - Fever
  - Rigors
  - Myalgia/arthralgias
- Psychiatric
  - Depression
  - Impaired concentration
  - Insomnia
  - Irritability
  - Mania
- Dermatologic
  - Pruritus
  - Dermatitis
  - Injection site reaction
  - Alopecia

- Gastrointestinal
  - Anorexia
  - Diarrhea
  - Nausea
  - Vomiting
- Pulmonary
  - Cough
  - Dyspnea
- Cytopenias
  - Thrombocytopenia
  - Hemolytic anemia
  - Leukopenia
- Other
  - Thyroid dysfunction
  - Ophthalmologic disorders (retinal hemorrhages)
  - Exacerbations of autoimmune diseases

Table 10.5 Dose Discontinuation/Reduction Rates

	IFN α-2b/RBV 1,000-1,200 mg (n = 505)	PEG-IFN α-2b 1.5/RBV 800 mg (n = 511)
Dose discontinuation for any adverse event	13%	14%
Dose reduction for:		
Adverse events	34%	42%
Anemia	13%	9%
Neutropenia	8%	18%
Thrombocytopenia	0%	0%
Depression	34%	31%

depression, psychosis, anxiety, insomnia, irritability, impaired concentration, and most importantly suicide, which can occur even after treatment has ended. The greatest risk factor for developing psychiatric symptoms on therapy is a prior psychiatric history. As psychiatric diagnoses are common in HCV, physicians should obtain a thorough psychiatric history prior to beginning HCV therapy. For patients found to have signs or symptoms, the treating clinician has several options. If the history shows only very minor issues, the patient may be able to be started on HCV therapy with close follow-up. If the history is more concerning, the clinician has the option of pretreating the patient with psychiatric medications (such as SSRI antidepressants) before starting HCV therapy or referring the patient to a psychologist/psychiatrist for formal evaluation and clearance. Whichever option is chosen, the patient ultimately needs close follow-up while on HCV therapy to monitor for worsening signs and symptoms of psychiatric illness.

Other major side effects include cytopenias. IFN can cause neutropenia and thrombocytopenia, while hemolytic anemia can be seen with RBV. Tables 10.6, 10.7, and 10.8 show package-insert management algorithms for the treatment of IFN-associated and RBV-associated anemia, neutropenia, and thrombocytopenia. Although not FDA approved for this indication, erythropoietin may be considered when Hgb levels drop in order to lessen the need for RBV

Table 10.6 PGN-IFN Alfa-2b Hematologic Dose Modification Guidelines

Laboratory Values	Dose Reduction	Discontinue if:
Hemoglobin decrease >2 g/dL in any 4-week period and stable cardiac disease	Decrease dose by 50%	Hemoglobin <12 g/dL after dose reductions
Hemoglobin <10 g/dL in patients without cardiac disease	Reduce dose by 50%	Hemoglobin <8.5 g/dL
WBC <1.5 × 10³/mm³, neutrophils < 0.75 × 10³/mm³, or platelets <50 × 10³/mm³	Reduce dose to 1 mcg/kg once weekly	WBC <1.0 × 10³/mm³, neutrophils <0.5 × 10³/mm³, or platelets <25 × 10³/mm³

Table 10.7 PGN-IFN Alfa-2a and Alfa-2b Hematological Dose Modification Guidelines

Laboratory Values	Dose Reduction	Discontinue if:
ANC < 750/mm³	135 mcg	ANC < 500 mm³ → D/C PEG-IFN alfa-2a and alfa-2b until ANC > 1,000 mm³, then restart at 90 mcg and monitor ANC
Platelets < 50,000/mm³	90 mcg	Platelet count < 25,000/mm³

dose reductions. In addition, filgrastim injections can be considered for the treatment of significant neutropenia to help lessen the need for IFN dose reductions.

In addition to the hemolytic anemia, there are some other issues specifically related to RBV. It is cleared by the kidney and caution should be used in patients with renal disease, as RBV levels rise and can cause worsening anemia. RBV is also a known teratogen, so strict contraception with two forms of birth control is necessary both during treatment and up to 6 months afterwards. This is true for both female and male patients.

On-Treatment Monitoring

Throughout therapy, HCV RNA levels are measured at standard intervals (4, 12, and 24 weeks) to predict response and guide length of therapy. The various definitions used in clinical practices are outlined in Table 10.9.

A rapid virologic response (RVR) is defined as a negative HCV RNA at 4 weeks and is highly predictive of achieving an SVR. Similar to SVR, RVR rates correlate with genotype. RVRs range from 15% to 20% in genotype 1 patients but are up to 66% in genotype 2 or 3 patients (Ferenci et al., 2005; Shiffman et al., 2007). Although less common in patients with genotype 1, those who achieved an RVR had a 91% chance of achieving an SVR (Ferenci et al., 2005).

Early virologic response (EVR) is evaluated at week 12 of therapy. An EVR can be complete or partial. A complete EVR is defined as HCV RNA negative at 12 weeks. A partial EVR is defined as a decrease in HCV RNA of more than 2 log (compared to baseline) at 12 weeks. For genotype 1 patients who achieve at least a partial EVR, 65% to 72% will ultimately achieve an SVR (Davis et al., 2003). If a complete EVR is achieved, treatment should be continued for 48 weeks. Failure to achieve at least a partial EVR is associated with an extremely low chance of SVR (1% to 3%) and is used by most investigators as a way to identify nonresponders and thus terminate therapy early (Fried et al., 2002; Manns et al., 2001). If patients achieve a partial EVR (but not a complete EVR),

Table 10.9 Definitions of Virologic Response to Antiviral Therapy for Hepatitis C	
Response	**Definition**
Rapid virologic response (RVR)	HCV RNA negative at 4 weeks as defined by HCV RNA <50 IU/mL
Early virologic response (cEVR)	HCV RNA negative or >2 $\log^{10}$ drop at week 12
End-of-treatment response (ETR)	HCV RNA negative at last dose of treatment regimen
Sustained virologic response (SVR)	HCV RNA negative 24 weeks after end of treatment

HCV RNA should be checked at 24 weeks, and if HCV RNA is still detectable at any level, treatment should then be discontinued.

Although the standard treatment is 48 weeks for genotype 1 patients and 24 weeks for genotype 2 and 3 patients, many investigators have examined shortening or lengthening therapy based on the on-treatment HCV viral kinetics. For example, in patients who achieve an RVR, shortening of treatment duration may be possible; however, relapse rates may be higher with a shortened treatment course. On the other hand, for patients who are responding more slowly to therapy, there has been a suggestion that lengthening treatment course up to 72 weeks may provide an opportunity to achieve an SVR. Whether this approach is reasonable or whether patients should be placed on the new direct-acting antiviral agents (described in a subsequent chapter) is open to debate. Figure 10.6 shows an algorithm that outlines some possible approaches to guide therapy duration in genotype 1 patients based on viral response (Marcellin et al., 2007).

Special Populations

Special considerations need to be made in several groups of patients both prior to and during treatment. These include patients co-infected with HIV, those with concomitant kidney disease, those of different ethnicities, and those who did not respond to previous HCV treatment regimens.

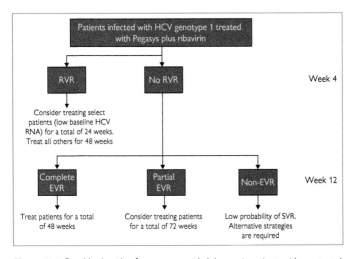

Figure 10.6 Possible algorithm for response-guided therapy in patients with genotype 1

Co-infection with HCV occurs in up to 30% of HIV-positive patients (Ghany et al., 2009). Because of recent advances in HIV therapy, patients are no longer dying as commonly of AIDS-related complications. Thus, a higher proportion of patients are now developing complications from end-stage liver disease. Patients co-infected with HIV and HCV will experience a faster progression of their liver disease. For these reasons, even though they have lower rates of SVR compared to patients with HCV alone, treatment should be considered in all co-infected patients. Many trials have looked at the treatment of HCV in HIV-positive patients. The largest trial, the APRICOT trial, used PEG-IFN + RBV and had SVR rates of 62% for patients with genotypes 2 and 3 and 29% for those with genotype 1 (Torriani et al., 2004). Based on the trial results, it has been recommended to treat patients with HIV/HCV co-infection with 48 weeks of PEG-IFN + RBV at the same doses used for HCV mono-infection. Patients with extremely low CD4 counts tend to have lower SVR rates, so ideally the patient's HIV should be treated and stabilized before therapy for HCV is introduced.

A second group of patients who need special consideration are those with kidney disease. Patients on hemodialysis have high rates of HCV infection and should be tested. Any patient with renal disease and HCV needs to be considered for treatment, as this group has an increased rate of progression to cirrhosis and development of HCC (Nakayama et al., 2000). RBV is completely cleared by the kidney and the clearance of IFN is also reduced in kidney disease, so special considerations are necessary when treating this class of patients. If the creatinine clearance exceeds 60 mL/min (CKD 1 or 2), treatment can be given at standard doses. For patients with CKD 3 to 5 (pre-hemodialysis), there are limited trials to give any definite recommendations. Some experts recommend avoiding (or at least severely limiting the use of) RBV in such patients. Other available guidelines suggest cautious use of both agents at reduced doses (Ghany et al., 2009). For patients with end-stage renal disease on dialysis, any HCV treatment should be given with extreme caution, and there should be close observation for side effects. Most experts would avoid the use of RBV in these dialysis patients.

African Americans have lower response rates to HCV therapy (Aronsohn & Reau, 2009). Two studies comparing African Americans to non-Hispanic whites with genotype 1 HCV found significantly lower rates of SVR in the African American group (19% to 28% vs. 52%) (Conjeevaram et al., 2006; Muir et al., 2004). A similar trend was seen in a separate study comparing African Americans and Caucasians with genotype 2 and 3 HCV (Shiffman et al., 2007). Despite these lower response rates, it is still recommended that African Americans with HCV should be treated with PEG-IFN + RBV at standard doses. Patients of Latino descent have also been shown to have lower rates of SVR when compared to Caucasians (Rodriguez-Torres et al., 2008).

The final group that needs special consideration is those who did not respond to their initial HCV therapy. These include patients who were either nonresponders (those who were never HCV RNA negative on treatment) or relapsers (those who were HCV RNA negative on therapy but relapsed after therapy was discontinued). There are several factors that predict a nonresponse or relapse, such as genotype, degree of liver fibrosis, dose of treatment (dose reductions in either the IFN or RBV are associated with higher rates of nonresponse), and patients' tolerance to and compliance with the initial treatment. Overall, using standard IFN and RBV, approximately 60% of treatment-naïve patients will not achieve an SVR (approximately 70% in genotype 1 patients and 35% in genotype 2 and 3 patients) (McHutchison & Poynard, 1999). For those receiving PEG-IFN + RBV as their initial therapy, 45% will not achieve SVR (approximately 55% in genotype 1 patients and 20% in genotype 2 and 3 patients) (Fried et al., 2002; Manns et al., 2001).

Several techniques have been attempted to retreat HCV patients who failed to respond to prior courses of therapy. For patients originally treated with standard IFN + RBV, retreatment with PEG-IFN + RBV can be attempted but is associated with limited success.

For patients who failed therapy with PEG-IFN + RBV, the treatment options are also quite limited. Retreatment with the same regimen is not recommended, as less than 5% will achieve an SVR with this method (Cheruvattath et al., 2007). Jensen et al. (2009) evaluated the use of double-dose PEG-IFN induction therapy and standard-dose RBV for 12 weeks followed by an additional 60 weeks of standard-dose PEG-IFN + RBV. The study did find a significantly increased SVR rate, but the 72-week group still had an SVR rate of only 16% (Jensen et al., 2009).

Another approach to the treatment of the previous nonresponders has been maintenance therapy using low-dose PEG-IFN without RBV. In the HALT-C study, previous nonresponders were randomized to receive either PEG-IFN alfa-2a at 90 µg/week for 3.5 years or no treatment. At the end of the study, a higher mortality and incidence of ascites were seen in the treatment group (Di Bisceglie et al., 2008). A second study, COPILOT, also looked at maintenance therapy in previous nonresponders. In this randomized, controlled, multicenter study, patients were given PEG-IFN alfa-2b 0.5 µg/kg per week or colchicine 0.6 mg orally, twice daily, over a treatment period of 4 years (Afdhal et al., 2008). At the conclusion of the study, there were no significant differences in primary endpoints, including event-free survival. Based on the above data, maintenance therapy is also not recommended.

Conclusion

HCV treatment with IFN-based therapy can be challenging and yet rewarding. SVR, the ultimate goal in HCV therapy, probably represents a cure of the infection and has been associated with improvements in overall patient outcomes. Significant advances in HCV therapy have been seen over the past two decades. When standard IFN monotherapy was introduced in the 1990s, SVR rates ranged from 0% to 10%. Currently, using PEG-IFN + RBV, overall SVR rates for HCV are approximately 55% (approximately 45% in genotype 1 patients and 80% in genotypes 2 and 3 patients).

Even though significant progress has been made in HCV treatment, there are still a considerable number of patients who will not respond to PEG-IFN + RBV therapy. Newer options will include combining PEG-IFN + RBV with direct-acting antiviral agents. These will be described in a subsequent chapter.

References

Afdhal, N., R. Levin, R. Brown Jr., et al. (2008). Colchicine versus peginterferon alfa 2b long term therapy: results of the 4 year COPILOT trial. *Journal of Hepatology, 48,* Abstract 3.

Armstrong, G. L., A. Wasley, E. P. Simard, et al. (2006). The prevalence of hepatitis C virus infection in the United States, 1999 through 2002. *Annals of Internal Medicine, 144,* 705–714.

Aronsohn, A., & N. Reau (2009). Long-term outcomes after treatment with interferon and ribavirin in HCV patients. *Journal of Clinical Gastroenterology, 43,* 661–671.

Backus, L. I., D. B. Boothroyd, B. R. Phillips, et al. (2011). A sustained virologic response reduces risk of all-cause mortality in patients with hepatitis C. *Clinical Gastroenterology & Hepatology, 9,* 509–516.

Centers for Disease Control and Prevention (2001). *Hepatitis C: National prevention strategy.* Retrieved from http://www.cdc.gov/hepatitis/HCV/Strategy/NatHepCPrevStrategy.htm

Cheruvattath, R., M. J. Rosati, M. Gautam, et al. (2007). Pegylated interferon and ribavirin failures: is retreatment an option? *Digestive Disease Science, 52,* 732–736.

Conjeevaram, H. S., M. W. Fried, L. J. Jeffers, et al. (2006). Peginterferon and ribavirin treatment in African Americans and Caucasian American patients with hepatitis C genotype 1. *Gastroenterology, 131,* 470–471.

Davis, G. L., J. B. Wong, J. B. McHutchison, et al. (2003). Early virologic response to treatment with peginterferon alfa-2b plus ribavirin in patients with chronic hepatitis C. *Hepatology, 38,* 645–652.

Di Bisceglie, A. M., M. L. Shiffman, G. T. Everson, et al. (2008). Prolonged therapy of advanced chronic hepatitis C with low-dose peginterferon. *New England Journal of Medicine, 359,* 2429–2441.

Ferenci, P., M. W. Fried, M. L. Shiffman, et al. (2005). Predicting sustained viroloical responses in chronic hepatitis C patients treated with peginterferon alfa-2a (40 KD)/ribavirin. *Journal of Hepatology, 43,* 425–433.

Finelli, L., J. T. Miller, J. I. Tokars, et al. (2005). National surveillance of dialysis-associated diseases in the United States. *Seminars Dialysis, 18,* 52–61.

Fried, M. W., M. L. Shiffman, K. R. Reddy, et al. (2002). Peginterferon alfa-2a plus ribavirin for chronic hepatitis C virus infection. *New England Journal of Medicine, 347,* 975–982.

Ge, D., J. Fellay, A. J. Thompson, et al. (2009). Genetic variation in IL28B predicts hepatitis C treatment-induced viral clearance. *Nature, 461,* 399–401.

Ghany, M. G., D. B. Strader, D. L. Thomas, & L. B. Seeff (2009). AASLD practice guidelines: Diagnosis, management, and treatment of hepatitis C: An update. *Hepatology, 49,* 1335–1374.

Hadziyannis, S. J., H. Sette Jr., T. R. Morgan, et al. (2004). Peginterferon-alpha2a and ribavirin combination therapy in chronic hepatitis C: a randomized study of treatment duration and ribavirin dose. *Annals of Internal Medicine, 140(5),* 346–355.

Heathcote, J., & J. Main. (2005). Treatment of hepatitis C. *Journal of Viral Hepatitis, 12,* 223–235.

Jensen, D. M., P. Marcellin, B. Freilich, et al. (2009). Re-treatment of patients with chronic hepatitis C who do not respond to peginterferon-alpha2b: a randomized trial. *Annals of Internal Medicine, 150,* 528–540.

Kim, A., & S. Saab (2005). Treatment of hepatitis C. *American Journal of Medicine, 118,* 808–815.

Lauer, G. M., & B. D. Walker (2001). Hepatitis C virus infection. *New England Journal of Medicine, 345,* 41–52.

Lindsay, K. (2002). Introduction to therapy of hepatitis C. *Hepatology, 36*(5) (Suppl. 1), S114–120.

Manns, M. P., J. G. McHutchison, S. C. Gordon, et al. (2001). Peginterferon alfa-2b plus ribavirin for initial treatment of chronic hepatitis C: a randomised trial. *Lancet, 358,* 958–965.

Marcellin, P., D. M. Jensen, S. J. Hadziyannis, et al. (2007). Differentiation of early virologic response (EVR) into RVR, complete EVR (cEVR) and partial EVR (pEVR) allows for a more precise prediction of SVR in genotype 1 patients treated with peginterferon alfa-2A (40 kD)(Pegasys) and ribavirin (Copegus). *Hepatology, 46,* 818A.

McHutchison, J. G., T. Poynard. (1999). Combination therapy with interferon plus ribavirin for the initial treatment of chronic hepatitis C. *Seminars Liver Disease, 19*(suppl 1), 57–65.

Muir, A. J., J. D. Bornstein, & P. G. Killenberg. (2004). Peginterferon alfa-2b and ribavirin for the treatment of chronic hepatitis C in blacks and non-Hispanic whites. *New England Journal of Medicine, 350,* 2265–2271.

Nakayama, E., T. Akiba, F. Marumo, & C. Sato (2000). Prognosis of anti-hepatitis C virus antibody-positive patients on regular hemodialysis therapy. *Journal of the American Society of Nephrology, 11,* 1896–1902.

National Institute of Health (2002). *Consensus development program: Management of hepatitis C.* Retrieved from http://consensus.nih.gov/2002/2002HepatitisC2002116html.htm

Rodriguez-Torres, M., L. J. Jeffers, M. Y. Sheikh, et al. (2008). Virologic responses to pegIFN-2a/ribavirin in treatment-naïve Latino verses non-Latino Caucasians infected with HCV genotype 1: the LATINO study. *Journal of Hepatology, 48*(s2), S311.

Shiffman, M. L., A. A. Mihas, F. Millwala, et al. (2007). Treatment of chronic hepatitis C virus in African Americans with genotypes 2 and 3. *American Journal of Gastroenterolgoy, 102,* 761–766.

Swain, M., M. Y. Lai, M. L. Shiffman, et al. (2010). A sustained virological response is a durable in patients with chronic hepatitis C treated with peginterferon alfa-2a and ribavirin. *Gastroenterology, 139*(5), 1593–1601.

Thomas, D. L., C. L. Thio, M. P. Martin, et al. (2009). Genetic variation in IL28B and spontaneous clearance of hepatitis C virus. *Nature, 461,* 798–802.

Torriani, F. J., M. Rodriguez-Torres, J. Rockstroh, et al. (2004). Peginterferon alfa-2a plus ribavirin for chronic hepatitis C virus infection in HIV-infected patients. *New England Journal of Medicine, 351,* 438–450.

Chapter 11

Side Effect Management of Peginterferon and Ribavirin

Christopher E. McGowan and Michael W. Fried

Virtually all patients treated with combination peginterferon (PEG-IFN) and ribavirin (RBV) for hepatitis C will experience a treatment-related side effect. Adverse events occur secondary to IFN, RBV, or the combination of both agents, and may reduce adherence to therapy, lead to suboptimal dosing, or result in treatment discontinuation. In the registration trials of PEG-IFN + RBV, 10% to 14% of patients discontinued therapy due to adverse events, with dose reductions occurring in 32% to 42% of patients (Fried et al., 2002; Manns et al., 2001). The most commonly experienced side effects are constitutional, hematologic (anemia, neutropenia, thrombocytopenia), and psychiatric (Table 11.1). The presentation and management of common treatment-related side effects will be discussed in this chapter. The novel adverse event profiles of the protease inhibitors telaprevir and boceprevir will be reviewed in Chapter 13.

General Considerations

The anticipation of treatment-related side effects represents a significant source of anxiety for patients considering antiviral therapy. Providers should hold a frank and thorough discussion of potential side effects with all patients, including their family members and caregivers. This discussion should be held prior to treatment initiation and should include a plan for monitoring and treating any side effects and symptoms that may develop. Patients should be advised to maintain adequate hydration and a light to moderate exercise program. Tailoring the dosing schedule to coincide with the patient's days off from work may be further beneficial. Each of these measures will help reduce patients' anxiety, prepare them for potential side effects, and improve adherence to therapy.

Patients should be evaluated at regular intervals during treatment so that side effects and symptoms can be promptly identified and managed. Providers should inquire specifically about constitutional symptoms (e.g., fatigue, fever, myalgias), dyspnea, visual disturbances, skin findings, and changes in mood. Routine laboratory testing should include a complete blood count at weeks 2 and 4, followed by every 4 to 8 weeks during treatment. Thyroid-stimulating hormone (TSH) and free thyroxine (free T4) should be measured at baseline and every 12 weeks during treatment. Further testing as well as referral

Table 11.1 Frequency of Side Effects Associated with PEG-IFN + RBV Combination Therapy

Side Effect	Frequency (%)
Fatigue	54–64
Headache	47–62
Myalgias	42–56
Pyrexia	43–46
Rigors	24–48
Insomnia	37–40
Nausea	29–43
Alopecia	28–36
Irritability	24–35
Arthralgias	27–34
Anorexia/weight loss	21–32
Depression	22–31
Dermatitis	21–24

Adapted from Fried, M. W., et al. (2002). *New England Journal of Medicine, 347*(13), 975–982; and Manns, M. P., et al. (2001). *Lancet, 358*(9286), 958–965.

for specialist input and management should be based on the development of particular symptoms or side effects, as discussed below. A summary of management recommendations for common side effects is presented in Table 11.2.

Constitutional Symptoms

Constitutional symptoms are the most frequently encountered side effects of therapy. Influenza-like symptoms, including fatigue, pyrexia, headache, myalgia, rigors, and arthralgias, are experienced by more than half of patients receiving PEG-IFN, with essentially all patients experiencing at least one of these symptoms within the first few doses (Fried et al., 2002; Manns et al., 2001). Fortunately, constitutional symptoms generally occur early during treatment (in the first few weeks) and tend to attenuate after 4 to 6 weeks of therapy. Acetaminophen or ibuprofen may prevent or reduce these symptoms when taken 30 minutes prior to PEG-IFN injection. All patients should be advised to maintain adequate hydration.

Hematologic Side Effects

Anemia

Anemia is a leading cause of treatment dose reduction and reduced quality of life in patients receiving combination PEG-IFN + RBV. The accumulation of RBV in red blood cells leads to increased oxidative damage and subsequent extravascular hemolysis. Additionally, IFN may impair hemoglobin production via bone marrow suppression, though this effect is less pronounced. In total,

Table 11.2 Recommendations for the Management of Common Side Effects of PEG-IFN + RBV Therapy

Fevers and chills	• Administer IFN at bedtime. • Pretreat with acetaminophen (1 gram) 30 minutes prior to interferon. • Patients should notify their provider if temperature is persistently >101°F.
Fatigue	• Administer IFN at bedtime. • Recommend low-impact exercise (i.e., walking, stretching). • If possible, reduce workload and/or take a short nap after work.
Insomnia	• Patient should take their second dose of RBV before 6 p.m. • Recommend good sleep habits (e.g., avoid TV in bed, limit caffeine). • Diphenhydramine 25 mg at bedtime may be helpful. • Prescription sleep aids (e.g., Ambien) where necessary
Muscle and body aches	• Acetaminophen (up to 2 grams daily) or NSAIDS (avoid if cirrhotic) • Follow a low-impact exercise plan. • Maintain adequate hydration (8–10 glasses of non-caffeinated fluid/day). • Apply warm moist heat (such as a warm washcloth).
Poor appetite	• Eat small, frequent meals (3 meals + 2 or 3 snacks per day). • Drink supplements (e.g., Carnation Instant Breakfast, Ensure). • Eat snacks with protein (cheese, peanut butter, eggs).
Nausea/vomiting	• Eat smaller meals; avoid smells and foods that trigger nausea. • Take RBV with food. • Ginger may be helpful (tea, ale, snaps). • Anti-emetics
Rash and pruritus	• Patients should wear sunscreen and avoid prolonged periods in the sun. • Avoid hot showers and vigorous rubbing of the skin; moisturize skin. • Topical low-dose steroid cream (1% hydrocortisone or triamcinolone) • Oral antihistamines (e.g., Benadryl, Allegra, Claritin, or Zyrtec) • Patients should notify their provider if blistering, widespread rash, or fever occurs.
Alopecia	• Use a wide-tooth comb. Avoid harsh hair products. • Hair loss is mild and typically reversible after treatment completion.
Vision changes	• Patients should contact their provider if visual changes develop. • Pretreatment ophthalmologic exam if diabetes, hypertension, or unilateral blindness
Depression, anxiety, irritability	• Patients should contact their provider with any changes in mood. • Consider SSRIs for depressive-specific symptoms. • Consider stimulants (methylphenidate or modafinil) for neurovegetative symptoms. • Patients with severe depression and/or suicidal ideation require treatment discontinuation and prompt psychiatric referral.

Adapted from Carol Pillsbury, MSN, NP-C, and Jama Darling, MD; UNC Liver Center, Chapel Hill, NC.

approximately one third of patients treated with combination therapy will develop anemia, with 9% to 15% of patients requiring a RBV dose reduction. The mean decrease in hemoglobin concentration is approximately 2.5 g/dL, typically occurring by treatment week 6 to 8 (Ghany et al., 2009).

Anemia may lead to fatigue and decreased quality of life, factors known to influence adherence to therapy. Therefore, dose reductions are necessary when anemia develops. In general, RBV dose reduction is recommended when the hemoglobin level falls below 10 g/dL, with discontinuation of therapy below 8.5 g/dL (Table 11.3) (Pegasys and Copegus prescribing information; PegIntron and Rebetol prescribing information). Retrospective studies have demonstrated that a hemoglobin drop of 1.5 g/dL at week 2 is highly predictive of subsequent development of more severe anemia (Reau et al., 2008). Thus, earlier, modest dose reductions of RBV by 200-mg decrements may obviate more drastic reductions or treatment discontinuation.

Recombinant erythropoietin (EPO) is frequently used to counter treatment-induced anemia, although it is not approved for this indication. The use of EPO has been shown to improve quality of life and reduce the need for RBV dose reduction. However, it has no proven benefit on sustained virologic response (SVR) (Ghany et al., 2009). EPO can be considered for patients who exhibit severe symptoms related to anemia, as well as in patients at risk of treatment discontinuation. EPO therapy can be initiated when the hemoglobin decreases below 10 g/dL (EASL guidelines, 2011). Response should be assessed after 2 weeks, with EPO discontinued if the hemoglobin increases by 1 g/dL or more. Otherwise, hemoglobin should be reassessed after 4 weeks, and EPO should be discontinued if the hemoglobin increases by 2 g/dL or more. If the hemoglobin exceeds 12 g/dL at any time, EPO should likewise be discontinued. Further monitoring and reinstitution of EPO may be necessary. In general, EPO is well tolerated, though known side effects include headache, nausea, arthralgias, and potential cardiovascular and thromboembolic events. More rarely, pure red cell aplasia may develop.

Neutropenia

Neutropenia, defined as an absolute neutrophil count (ANC) below 750/mm^3, is a common hematologic side effect of IFN use and a frequent reason for dose reduction. Neutropenia occurs in approximately 20% of patients treated with combination PEG-IFN + RBV. A rapid decline in ANC, generally 30% to 50% from baseline, can be expected in the first 2 weeks of therapy, with counts usually stabilizing over the subsequent 4 to 6 weeks (Mac Nicholas & Norris, 2010). Importantly, blood counts should be measured the day before, rather than the day after, IFN dosing so as to best estimate nadir hematologic parameters.

If neutropenia develops during therapy, patients should be monitored weekly until counts stabilize. The major concern with neutropenia is the development of infectious complications. Fortunately, the decline in ANC is usually not associated with an increased risk of infection. Prospective studies have maintained full PEG-IFN dosing with ANC levels between 250 and 500/mm^3 without adverse infectious complications (Conjeevaram et al., 2006). Nevertheless, reduction of the PEG-IFN dose should be considered in the presence of neutropenia (see Table 11.3) (Pegasys and Copegus prescribing

Table 11.3 Recommended Dose Adjustments for Hematologic Complications of PEG-IFN + RBV Combination Therapy

Laboratory Parameter	PEG-IFN alfa-2a (PEGASYS) and RBV (COPEGUS)	PEG-IFN alfa-2b (PegIntron) and RBV (REBETOL)
Neutrophil Count		
<0.75 × 10³/mm³	Reduce PEGASYS to 135 mcg/week.	Reduce PegIntron dose by half.
<0.5 × 10³/mm³	Suspend PEGASYS until ANC >1.0, then resume at 90 mcg/week.	Discontinue therapy.
Platelet Count		
<50 × 10³/mm³	Reduce PEGASYS to 90 mcg/week.	Reduce PegIntron dose by half.
<25 × 10³/mm³	Discontinue therapy.	Discontinue therapy.
Hemoglobin		
<10 g/dL*	Reduce COPEGUS to 600 mg/day.	Reduce REBETOL by 200 mg/day.
<8.5 g/dL	Discontinue therapy.	Discontinue therapy.

*For patients with a history of stable cardiac disease, dose reduction to 600 mg/day (COPEGUS) or by 200 mg/day (REBETOL) is recommended for any 2-g/dL or greater decrease in hemoglobin during any 4-week period.

Adapted from PEGASYS/COPEGUS prescribing information (Genentech; available at http://www.gene.com/gene/products/information/pegasys) and PegIntron/REBETOL prescribing information (Merck; available at http://www.spfiles.com/pipeg-intron.pdf).

information; PegIntron and Rebetol prescribing information). White blood cell counts rapidly return to baseline after treatment discontinuation, and IFN can be restarted when the ANC improves to 1,000/mm³, though at a reduced dosage. There is no evidence that granulocyte colony-stimulating factor (G-CSF) improves sustained response rates or reduces infectious complications of neutropenia in HCV patients; therefore, routine use is not currently recommended (Ghany et al., 2009).

Thrombocytopenia

A decrease in platelet count is common with IFN therapy, resulting from reduced thrombopoietin production and/or increased platelet sequestration. A 10% to 50% decrease in platelet count can be expected; however, only 4% of patients will require a dose reduction of IFN (Russo & Fried, 2003). Bleeding complications are rare. The decrease in platelet count is generally sustained during treatment and resolves upon completion. Though rarely a problem in most patients, thrombocytopenia may be a significant concern in patients with underlying cirrhosis and portal hypertension, where preexisting thrombocytopenia is often present. In these patients, the risk of a further decrease in platelet count may preclude treatment initiation. For patients who develop thrombocytopenia during treatment, dose reduction is recommended when the platelet count falls below 75,000/mm³ (see Table 11.3) (Pegasys and Copegus prescribing information; PegIntron and Rebetol prescribing information). Complete discontinuation may be necessary if counts decline further. The use of thrombopoietin mimetics has been investigated, though their routine use is not currently recommended (McHutchinson et al., 2007). Immune-mediated thrombocytopenia, causing profound thrombocytopenia, may also complicate IFN therapy. This complication is rare and generally responds to withdrawal of treatment and initiation of corticosteroids, if necessary.

Neuropsychiatric Side Effects

Neuropsychiatric side effects are frequent in patients treated for hepatitis C and include fatigue, irritability, anxiety, and mood disorders (Evon et al., 2009). The development of neuropsychiatric side effects may have a negative impact on quality of life and treatment adherence; therefore, all patients should undergo a mental health assessment prior to initiating antiviral therapy. The most significant risk factor for the development of on-treatment neuropsychiatric side effects is their presence prior to treatment, underscoring the importance of early screening and identification. Further risk factors include younger age, less education, unemployment, poor social support, and single relationship status. The majority of neuropsychiatric side effects develop within the first 12 weeks of therapy, and are generally divided into two distinct syndromes: neurovegetative (including fatigue, psychomotor slowing, and anorexia) and depressive-specific (including depressed mood, anhedonia, anxiety, and subjective cognitive disturbance). The management of these syndromes differs (Raison et al., 2005).

In the pivotal PEG-IFN studies, depression was the most frequent reason for treatment discontinuation, reported in 22% to 31% of patients (Fried et al., 2002; Manns et al., 2001). Fortunately, depressive-specific symptoms are highly responsive to antidepressants, in particular the selective serotonin reuptake inhibitors (SSRIs). When selecting an antidepressant, clinicians should consider the patient's symptomatology, with particular SSRIs being more activating (e.g., fluoxetine and sertraline) and others less activating (e.g., paroxetine and fluvoxamine). Additionally, drug–drug interactions and potential hepatotoxicity should be considered. The tricyclic antidepressants should generally be avoided given their tendency toward sedation. For patients at high risk of developing depressive symptoms, antidepressant therapy may be initiated prophylactically, prior to treatment initiation. Otherwise, patients should be regularly assessed during treatment for the presence of depression, with initiation of an SSRI should it develop. Patients with severe depressive symptoms, including suicidal ideation, should receive immediate psychiatric consultation and IFN therapy should be promptly discontinued in these patients. Additionally, patients who fail to respond to antidepressant therapy may warrant psychiatric consultation. Finally, the development of mania, though rare, requires prompt psychiatric referral.

Neurovegetative symptoms are common, with fatigue occurring in 48% to 64% of patients (Fried et al., 2002; Manns et al., 2001). Importantly, these symptoms generally do not respond to treatment with SSRIs. Patients with these symptoms (and absence of depressive-specific findings) may benefit from agents that augment noradrenergic and dopaminergic function, such as the antidepressant bupropion. Psychostimulants, such as methylphenidate and modafinil, have been rarely used.

It is worth noting that with a multidisciplinary approach to the management of neuropsychiatric side effects, including adequate pretreatment and on-treatment evaluation, patients can be expected to achieve SVR rates comparable to those in persons without these complications.

Thyroid Side Effects

Up to 15% of patients treated with IFN may develop clinically significant thyroid disease, including hyperthyroidism or hypothyroidism (Mandac et al., 2006). The immunomodulatory properties of IFN may contribute to the development of Graves' disease, Hashimoto's thyroiditis, or asymptomatic thyroid antibodies. Non-autoimmune processes, including destructive thyroiditis, may also occur.

All patients should be screened for thyroid disease with a serum TSH and free T4 prior to treatment initiation, every 12 weeks during treatment, and after completion of therapy. Patients with pretreatment thyroid antibodies are at greater risk of developing thyroid disease; however, the routine measurement of autoantibodies is unlikely to alter management decisions. All patients should be assessed at each visit for symptoms of thyroid dysfunction, including excessive fatigue, weight loss or gain, hair loss, and heat or cold intolerance. These symptoms may be inappropriately attributed to IFN therapy or HCV infection; therefore, clinicians need to maintain a high index of suspicion. This will prevent delays in diagnosis and treatment.

For patients diagnosed with hypothyroidism, thyroid hormone replacement can be administered without the need to discontinue antiviral therapy. Serum TSH should be monitored at 2-month intervals, with hormone replacement adjusted accordingly. Endocrinology referral is recommended for patients who develop hyperthyroidism. Following IFN therapy, improvement in thyroid function may be observed in some patients.

Respiratory Side Effects

Patients treated with combination therapy may experience a nonproductive, persistent cough attributed to RBV, reported in up to one quarter of patients. Severe pulmonary toxicity from PEG-IFN is rare and includes interstitial pneumonitis, bronchiolitis obliterans with organizing pneumonia (BOOP), and the development or exacerbation of sarcoidosis (Slavenburg et al., 2010). All patients with persistent cough and dyspnea should be evaluated with a chest radiograph. Though rare, interstitial pneumonitis may be severe and even life-threatening; fortunately, it improves with withdrawal of therapy in most cases. The presence of sarcoidosis is generally considered a contraindication to IFN therapy, although individual benefits and risks for a specific patient must be considered. Treatment discontinuation may be necessary for patients who develop sarcoidosis during treatment.

Ophthalmologic Side Effects

Retinopathy is a common complication of IFN therapy, developing in nearly half of treated patients (Willson, 2004). Findings on funduscopic examination may include retinal hemorrhages and cotton-wool spots, though in general these changes are not associated with visual loss. Cotton-wool spots may be evanescent and do not require treatment discontinuation unless concomitant visual changes develop. Patients with underlying diabetes and hypertension are at increased risk of developing retinopathy and should be referred for a pre-treatment ophthalmologic examination. Likewise, an ophthalmologist should evaluate any patient who develops visual changes while receiving IFN therapy. In the setting of worsening retinopathy, IFN may need to be discontinued.

Dermatologic Side Effects

Dermatologic side effects occur in 21% to 24% of patients treated with combination PEG-IFN + RBV therapy (Fried et al., 2002; Manns et al., 2001). Findings may include generalized pruritus, skin xerosis, and eczematous lesions, usually attributed to RBV (Lubbe et al., 2005). These changes typically occur on extensor surfaces of the extremities and on truncal sites exposed to friction. They are distinct from IFN injection site reactions, which are experienced by one quarter of patients. Treatment of dermatitis involves the regular use of topical emollients and the intermittent use of a low- to moderate-potency topical corticosteroid. Oral antihistamines may provide additional relief. Dermatitis resolves after treatment cessation and rarely requires a dose reduction or treatment discontinuation. Hair loss is experienced by 28% to 36% of patients treated with combination therapy and includes telogen effluvium (loss of hair due to early entry into the telogen phase), localized injection site alopecia, and alopecia areata (Kartal et al., 2007). Patients should be reassured that these changes are usually mild and reversible after treatment completion.

Summary

All patients treated with PEG-IFN and RBV will experience adverse events associated with therapy. Educating the patient about expectations and self-management techniques and providing vigilant monitoring by clinicians will mitigate their impact on adherence and optimize treatment outcomes.

References

Conjeevaram, H. S., M. W. Fried, L. J. Jeffers, et al. (2006). PEG-IFN and RBV treatment in African American and Caucasian American patients with hepatitis C genotype 1. *Gastroenterology, 131*(2), 470–477.

(2011). EASL clinical practice guidelines: Management of hepatitis C virus infection. *Journal of Hepatology, 55*(2), 245–264.

Evon, D. M., D. Ramcharran, S. H. Belle, N. A. Terrault, R. J. Fontana, & M. W. Fried (2009). Prospective analysis of depression during PEG-IFN and RBV therapy of chronic hepatitis C: results of the Virahep-C study. *American Journal of Gastroenterology, 104*(12), 2949–2958.

Fried, M. W., M. L. Shiffman, K. R. Reddy, et al. (2002). PEG-IFN alfa-2a plus RBV for chronic hepatitis C virus infection. *New England Journal of Medicine 347*(13), 975–982.

Ghany, M. G., D. B. Strader, D. L. Thomas, & L. B. Seeff (2009). Diagnosis, management, and treatment of hepatitis C: an update. *Hepatology, 49*(4), 1335–1374.

Kartal, E. D., S. N. Alpat, I. Ozgunes, & G. Usluer (2007). Reversible alopecia universalis secondary to PEG-interferon alpha-2b and RBV combination therapy in a patient with chronic hepatitis C virus infection. *European Journal of Gastroenterolgoy & Hepatology, 19*(9), 817–820.

Lubbe, J., K. Kerl, F. Negro, & J. H. Saurat (2005). Clinical and immunological features of hepatitis C treatment-associated dermatitis in 36 prospective cases. *British Journal of Dermatology, 153*(5), 1088–1090.

Mac Nicholas, R., & S. Norris S. (2010). Review article: optimizing SVR and management of the haematological side effects of PEG-IFN/RBV antiviral therapy for HCV—the role of epoetin, G-CSF and novel agents. *Alimentary Pharmacology & Therapeutics, 31*(9), 929–937.

Mandac, J. C., S. Chaudhry, K. E. Sherman, & Y. Tomer (2006). The clinical and physiological spectrum of interferon-alpha induced thyroiditis: toward a new classification. *Hepatology, 43*(4), 661–672.

Manns, M. P., J. G. McHutchison, S. C. Gordon SC, et al. (2001). PEG-IFN alfa-2b plus RBV compared with interferon alfa-2b plus RBV for initial treatment of chronic hepatitis C: a randomised trial. *Lancet, 358*(9286), 958–965.

McHutchison, J. G., G. Dusheiko, M. L. Shiffman, et al. (2007). Eltrombopag for thrombocytopenia in patients with cirrhosis associated with hepatitis C. *New England Journal of Medicine, 357*(22), 2227–2236.

Pegasys and Copegus full prescribing information. http://www.gene.com/gene/products/information/pegasys. Accessed June 1, 2011.

PegIntron and Rebetol full prescribing information. http://www.spfiles.com/pipegintron.pdf. Accessed June 1, 2011.

Raison, C. L., M. Demetrashvili, L. Capuron, & A. H. Miller (2005). Neuropsychiatric adverse effects of interferon-alpha: recognition and management. *CNS Drugs, 19*(2), 105–123.

Reau, N., S. J. Hadziyannis, D. Messinger, M. W. Fried, & D. M. Jensen (2008). Early predictors of anemia in patients with hepatitis C genotype 1 treated with PEG-IFN alfa-2a (40KD) plus RBV. *American Journal of Gastroenterology, 103*(8), 1981–1988.

Russo, M. W., & M. W. Fried (2003). Side effects of therapy for chronic hepatitis C. *Gastroenterology, 124*(6), 1711–1719.

Slavenburg, S., Y. F. Heijdra, & J. P. Drenth (2010). Pneumonitis as a consequence of (peg)interferon-RBV combination therapy for hepatitis C: a review of the literature. *Digestive Disease Science, 55*(3), 579–585.

Willson, R. A. (2004). Visual side effects of pegylated interferon during therapy for chronic hepatitis C infection. *Journal of Clinical Gastroenterology, 38*(8), 717–722.

Chapter 12

Hepatitis C in Special Populations

Andres F. Carrion, Christin M. Giordano, and Paul Martin

Infection with the hepatitis C virus (HCV) remains responsible for approximately 40% of all cases of chronic liver disease in the United States and is the leading indication for liver transplantation in adults (Ghany et al., 2009). HCV represents a major public health problem, with an estimated prevalence of chronic infection of 1.6% in the U.S. population, although this is probably an underestimate. Infected individuals with specific challenges in management include those with chronic kidney disease (CKD), co-infection with human immunodeficiency virus (HIC), cirrhosis, ethnic minorities such as individuals of Hispanic and African American background, and elderly patients. Important differences exist in the epidemiology, natural history, eligibility for treatment, and outcomes for these subgroups when compared to the general population. This chapter addresses management of HCV infection in these key populations (Table 12.1). Although the advent of direct acting antiviral agents (DAAs) will profoundly alter the management of HCV, there are particular considerations in some of the populations we discuss to suggest that DAA therapy requires further study before it can be extended to all patients with chronic HCV.

Hepatitis C in Patients with CKD

Case: A 48-year-old Caucasian man is evaluated for management of treatment-naïve chronic hepatitis C (genotype 2a) infection. He has well-controlled systemic hypertension, stage III CKD (serum creatinine 2.3 mg/dL, creatinine clearance 33 mL/min/1.73 m^2), and anemia of chronic disease (hemoglobin 10.8 g/dL). There is no clinical evidence of decompensated liver disease. Liver biopsy reveals grade 1, stage 2 disease. Are there any particular considerations in considering anti-HCV therapy for this patient with renal disease?

The prevalence of HCV infection in patients with CKD receiving renal replacement therapy in the United States is higher than in the general population (7.5% to 14% vs. 1.6%, respectively) (Ghany et al., 2009). Nosocomial transmission within hemodialysis units, reflecting spread by interpersonal contact and contaminated medical supplies, is now the most important risk factor for HCV infection in this population. The risk of infection is proportional to the prevalence of HCV within individual hemodialysis units and time on hemodialysis (Fabrizi et al., 2002).

Table 12.1 Major Characteristics of HCV Infection in Special Populations

HCV in patients with CKD	• Higher prevalence than in non-CKD patients
	• HCV is associated with increased morbidity and mortality.
	• Decreased post-renal transplant patient and allograft survival
	• RBV-induced anemia is a major dose-limiting toxicity.
	• SVR with standard IFN monotherapy in patients on hemodialysis: 39%.
Recurrent HCV after liver transplantation	• Recurrent HCV occurs invariably and diminishes patient and allograft survival.
	• IFN may induce acute allograft rejection.
	• IFN and RBV improve patient and allograft survival when histologically significant recurrence is present.
	• Overall SVR with PEF-IFN and RBV: 30%
HCV and HIV co-infection	• HCV is the most common cause of liver-related death in patients with HIV.
	• HCV/HIV co-infection is associated with twofold greater risk of cirrhosis and sixfold greater risk of liver failure.
	• Successful treatment of HCV reduces liver decompensation, mortality, and HAART-induced hepatotoxicity.
	• RBV-induced anemia occurs frequently when zidovudine is used concomitantly.
	• The combination of RBV and didanosine is associated with severe toxicity.
	• Overall SVR with PEG-IFN and RBV: 40%
HCV in patients with cirrhosis	• Successful anti-HCV therapy results in histologic improvement, decreased incidence of clinical decompensation, and reduced risk of HCC.
	• In patients with compensated cirrhosis, SVR is 30% to 44%.
	• Anti-HCV therapy in decompensated cirrhosis is associated with significant toxicity.
HCV in ethnic minorities	• HCV is more prevalent in African American and Hispanic individuals in the United States.
	• Genotype 1 is found in 97% of African Americans with HCV.
	• SVR is lower for all genotypes in African American and Hispanic individuals using PEG-IFN and RBV.
	• The prevalence of the C/C gentoype of *IL28B* (favorable response to IFN-based therapy) is lower in African American than in Hispanic and NHW patients.
	• Boceprevir and telaprevir incrase SVR in African American patients.
HCV in elderly patients	• Lower prevalence of HCV compared to younger adults
	• Faster progression to fibrosis when infection occurs at older age
	• Elderly patients are less likely to be considered candidates for anti-HCV therapy.
	• Older age *per se* is not a contraindication for anti-HCV therapy.
	• Special attention should be given to comorbid conditions and medication-related side effects.

Current practice guidelines recommend testing for HCV in patients with CKD regardless of the severity of kidney disease in part because HCV infection can cause glomerulonephritis. Screening by now-standard third-generation enzyme immunoassay (EIA) is accurate in patients with CKD. Polymerase chain reaction (PCR) for HCV-ribonucleic acid (RNA) is used to detect viremia in seropositive patients and to exclude a false-negative antibody result if suspicion of HCV infection remains. Patients receiving maintenance hemodialysis should have monthly screening for HCV with alanine-aminotransferase (ALT) levels and biannual or yearly testing with EIA or PCR. Importantly, ALT levels may be well within the normal range in viremic patients on hemodialysis. If there is particular concern about HCV infection despite anti-HCV seronegativity (i.e., a patient undergoing hemodialysis in a unit with high prevalence of HCV or a renal transplant recipient with unexplained hepatic dysfunction), PCR testing for HCV-RNA should be obtained (Table 12.2) (Ghany et al., 2009; Kidney disease, 2008).

Hepatitis C in patients with CKD is associated with increased morbidity and mortality compared to noninfected patients with similar impairment of renal function. This difference may reflect faster progression to cirrhosis, with a higher incidence of hepatocellular carcinoma (HCC) (Fabrizi et al., 2004). Compared to HCV-negative renal transplant recipients, HCV-infected recipients have inferior patient and allograft survival rates. Furthermore, HCV is associated with multiple complications in the post-renal transplant period, including allograft nephropathy, new-onset diabetes after transplantation, and sepsis (Fabrizi et al., 2005).

Table 12.2 Diagnostic Recommendations for HCV in Patients with CKD

Population	Testing
CKD patients (no dialysis)	Test all patients, regardless of CKD stage, with third-generation EIA.
Initiation of hemodialysis	Third-generation EIA followed by PCR for HCV-RNA if positive
Transfer from hemodialysis unit with low prevalence of HCV	Third-generation EIA followed by PCR for HCV-RNA if positive
Transfer from hemodialysis unit with high prevalence of HCV	PCR for HCV-RNA
Hemodialysis at unit with low prevalence of HCV	Third-generation EIA every 6 to 12 months and monthly ALT
Hemodialysis at unit with high prevalence of HCV	PCR for HCV-RNA every 6 to 12 months and monthly ALT
Hemodialysis patients with unexplained abnormal ALT levels	PCR for HCV-RNA
Pre- and post-renal transplant periods	PCR for HCV-RNA
Suspicion of nosocomial infection or HCV outbreak at hemodialysis unit	PCR for HCV-RNA; retest in 2 to 12 weeks if negative

From Fabrizi et al., 2002; Ghany et al., 2009; Kidney Disease, 2008.

Current practice guidelines suggest consideration of anti-HCV therapy in patients with CKD who are candidates for renal transplantation and have an estimated survival of at least 5 years. It may also be appropriate to treat renal transplant candidates with CKD even when the pattern of histologic liver injury does not meet the standards for therapy in the general population (i.e., a METAVIR score ≥2/4 or an Ishak score ≥3/6 [Table 12.3]) (Ghany et al., 2009). Combination therapy with pegylated interferon (PEG-IFN) and ribavirin (RBV) at doses used in patients with intact renal function is recommended for patients with creatinine clearance 60 mL/min/1.73 m^2 and above (CKD stages 1 and 2). RBV is generally not recommended for patients with creatinine clearance below 50 mL/min/1.73 m^2; however, some data have suggested improved sustained virologic response (SVR) rates, defined by negative HCV-RNA 24 weeks after cessation of treatment, using combination therapy in this population (Rendina et al., 2007). Therefore, the guidelines recommend considering the combination of PEG-IFN (alfa-2a at 135 µg/week, or alfa-2b at 1 µg/kg/week) and RBV (200 to 800 mg/day divided in two doses) for patients not requiring dialysis with a creatinine clearance below 60 mL/min/1.73 m^2 (CKD stages 3, 4, and 5) (Ghany et al., 2009). Patients with CKD undergoing hemodialysis may be candidates for monotherapy with standard IFN alfa-2a or alfa-2b (3 million units thrice weekly). With this regimen, SVR is achieved in approximately 39% of patients, although approximately 19% of patients discontinue therapy due to side effects (Fabrizi et al., 2008). The addition of low doses of RBV to standard IFN in patients with CKD on hemodialysis may also result in higher SVR rates, but RBV-induced hemolytic anemia is an important dose-limiting toxicity. Therefore, close monitoring for side effects is mandatory when RBV is used in this population who has anemia at baseline, and dose reductions and/ or use of erythroid-stimulating agents (i.e., erythropoietin) may be necessary (Table 12.4).

Table 12.3 Scoring Systems for Histologic Stage of Fibrosis

Stage	METAVIR	Ishak
0	No fibrosis	No fibrosis
1	Periportal fibrotic expansion without septa	Fibrous expansion of some portal areas with or without short fibrous septa
2	Periportal septa	
3	Porto-central septa without cirrhosis	Fibrous expansion of most portal areas with occasional portal-to-portal bridging
4	Cirrhosis	Fibrous expansion of most portal areas with marked bridging (portal-to-portal and portal-to-central)
5		Marked bridging (portal-to-portal and portal-to-central) with occasional nodules (incomplete cirrhosis)
6		Cirrhosis

Ghany et al., 2009.

Table 12.4 Therapeutic Regimens Recommended for Treatment of HCV in Patients with Different Stages of CKD

CKD Stage	Creatinine Clearance (mL/min/1.73 m^2)	Recommended Anti-HCV Therapy
1	≥90	PEG-IFN + RBV
2	60–90	
3	30–59	PEG-IFN alfa-2b (1 µg/kg) or alfa-2a (135 µg) weekly plus RBV 200–800 mg/day divided in two doses
4	15–29	
5	<15	
5-D	<15 on hemodialysis	Standard IFN (alfa-2a or -2b) 3 million units thrice weekly (preferred regimen). Alternative: PEG-IFN alfa-2b 1 µg/kg/week, or PEG-IFN alfa-2a 135 µg/week ± very low dose RBV

Ghany et al., 2009.

Recently licensed DAAs such as boceprevir and telaprevir significantly improve SVR when used in combination with PEG-IFN and RBV. However, there are no data on treatment outcomes or toxicity associated with these drugs in patients with impaired renal function, and anemia remains an important concern due to required concomitant use of RBV. Data from key clinical trials of boceprevir and telaprevir in combination with PEG-IFN and RBV in patients with normal renal function indicate that the incidence of anemia was higher compared to PEG-IFN and RBV (37% to 49% vs. 19% to 29%, respectively). This suggests that use of these new agents will be difficult in patients with anemia due to CKD (Bacon et al., 2011;Jacobson et al., 2011; Poordad et al., 2011).

In conclusion, HCV infection in patients with CKD results in diminished survival due to hepatic complications and also impairs recipient and allograft survival following renal transplantation. The benefits of successful anti-HCV therapy are substantial in patients with CKD, including reducing the likelihood of allograft injury following renal transplantation. However, anti-HCV therapy is associated with significant toxicity in this population and it should be used only in patients without major comorbidities and a predicted reasonable long-term survival. The patient in the clinical vignette may be a candidate for therapy with PEG-IFN and low-dose RBV at an experienced center. Exacerbation of baseline anemia is a significant concern, requiring vigilant monitoring, erythroid-stimulating agents, and, if necessary, reduction of the RBV dosage.

Recurrent Hepatitis C after Liver Transplantation

Case: A 64-year-old Caucasian man underwent orthotopic liver transplantation 1 year ago for decompensated cirrhosis due to HCV infection with genotype 2b. The patient has had persistently elevated aminotransferases, with serial liver biopsies showing chronic inflammation without definitive evidence of rejection. The most recent biopsy also showed grade 2, stage 2 disease. The patient has not received anti-HCV therapy to date; tacrolimus is the only current immuno-suppressive. There are no other significant comorbidities. What is the role of antiviral therapy in this patient?

Hepatitis C is the leading indication for liver transplantation in adults in the United States. Recurrent hepatitis C occurs almost invariably in the allograft with an accelerated course, resulting in decreased patient and allograft survival (Rowe et al., 2008). Cirrhosis and overt decompensation due to recurrent HCV occur in approximately one third of patients within 5 years post-transplant, rising to 50% after 10 years. Recurrent HCV is responsible overall for 25% to 30% of all hepatic allograft losses (Forman et al., 2002).

Anti-HCV therapy in the post-liver transplant period presents some unique challenges. Liver transplant recipients typically require a variety of medications, including immunosuppressive, antihypertensive, and glucose-lowering agents. Renal insufficiency is also frequent and often progressive due to a variety of factors, including calcineurin-inhibitor (tacrolimus and cyclosporine) nephro-toxicity. This in turn results in anemia, adding to the complexity of using IFN and RBV post-liver transplantation. For instance, RBV-induced hemolytic ane-mia is the most commonly reported cause of treatment interruption in liver transplant recipients (Carrion et al., 2007). Hypersplenism due to portal hyper-tension can persist post-transplant, preventing adequate dosing of IFN and RBV due to hematologic toxicities. Immunosuppression increases HCV viral load often in a logarithmic fashion compared to pretransplant levels. Cirrhosis decreases tolerance for IFN because of medication-related side effects, there-fore resulting in frequent dropouts and lower SVR. Because of these concerns, less than half of liver transplant recipients with recurrent HCV infection are currently considered appropriate candidates for anti-HCV therapy.

IFN-induced acute allograft rejection is an important concern following solid-organ transplantation other than liver. Therefore, IFN-based therapy for HCV is currently contraindicated following heart, lung, and kidney transplanta-tion, except in recipients with post-transplant fibrosing cholestatic hepatitis as a desperate measure to preserve hepatic function (Ghany et al., 2009; Kidney Disease, 2008). In contrast, anti-HCV therapy with IFN-based regimens is not contraindicated in liver transplant recipients as allograft rejection, although a theoretical concern, has not been a major limitation in treatment. However, antiviral therapy following liver transplantation should be managed by experi-enced transplant providers (Stravitz et al., 2004).

Information on treatment strategies for recurrent HCV following liver transplantation is relatively limited and often based on small studies. Preemptive anti-HCV therapy peri-transplant and early post-transplant is not recom-mended due to lack of proven benefit in enhancing patient or allograft survival. Furthermore, this strategy results in frequent adverse effects, limiting effec-tive dosing (Craxi, 2011; Ghany et al., 2009). Most centers reserve antiviral therapy for recipients with established recurrent HCV infection, typically at least several months following transplantation. PEG-IFN alfa with RBV remains the typical regimen in liver transplant recipients with evidence of histologically significant recurrence (conventionally METAVIR stage ≥2/4 or Ishak stage ≥3/6) (Ghany et al., 2009). Unlike preemptive therapy, successful antiviral treatment in liver transplant recipients with fibrosis results in improved patient and allograft survival. In general, treatment with IFN-based regimens and RBV in liver transplant recipients with recurrent HCV yields SVR rates of approximately 30%. Importantly, the usual predictors of response, including specific genotype and on-treatment viral response, are also valid post-liver transplantation (Craxi, 2011).

In conclusion, recurrent hepatitis C after liver transplantation diminishes patient and allograft survival. Preemptive early post-transplant treatment, before HCV recurrence is established, is currently not recommended. However, successful anti-HCV therapy in post-liver transplant patients with significant fibrosis improves survival and should be attempted in the absence of major contraindications to therapy. The patient described above should be offered antiviral therapy as he already has stage 2 fibrosis.

Hepatitis C and HIV Co-infection

Case: A 38-year-old Caucasian woman with HIV infection diagnosed 8 years ago is evaluated for HCV infection. HIV is well controlled with highly active antiretroviral therapy (CD4+ 800/µL and undetectable HIV-RNA). She has no other medical comorbidities, serum aminotransferases are normal, and there is no evidence of decompensated liver disease. She has HCV genotype 1a, HCV-RNA load is 12,500,000 IU/mL, and liver biopsy shows grade 3, stage 2 disease. What is the role of anti-HCV therapy?

In the United States, approximately 8% of patients with hepatitis C are co-infected with HIV, and a higher proportion of HIV-infected patients have serologic evidence of HCV co-infection (20%). Co-infection with hepatitis B virus (HBV) occurs in 4.5% to 8% of HIV-infected patients in the United States, and triple infection with HCV and HBV in HIV-infected patients is not rare (1.6%) (Kim et al., 2008; Spradling et al., 2010). Co-infection reflects shared routes of transmission; therefore, patients infected with any of these viruses (HCV, HBV, or HIV) should be screened for co-infection. Approximately 1.8% of patients with HCV/HIV co-infection are anti-HCV seronegative when third-generation EIA tests are compared to HCV-RNA PCR. Therefore, it is important to exclude HCV viremia in HIV-infected patients with unexplained hepatic dysfunction despite negative HCV serologies (Bonacini et al., 2001).

Progression from acute to chronic HCV infection occurs more frequently in patients co-infected with HIV than in mono-infected patients. Approximately 92% to 95% of patients co-infected with HIV do not clear HCV following acute infection and develop chronic infection, in contrast to 70% to 85% of HIV-negative controls (Thomas et al., 2000). Furthermore, co-infection with HCV/HIV is associated with higher HCV-RNA levels, a twofold greater risk of progression to cirrhosis, and a sixfold greater risk of liver failure compared to HCV mono-infection (Graham et al., 2001). Liver disease is the most frequent non-AIDS-related cause of death in HIV-infected patients, with HCV infection being the most common etiology (66.1%), followed by HBV (16.9%) and HCV/HBV co-infection (7.1%) (Weber et al., 2006). The risk of HCC is fivefold higher among patients with co-infection and may occur at a younger age and with a shorter duration of HCV infection, and has a more aggressive course than in HIV-negative patients (Giordano et al., 2004; Matthews & Dore, 2008). Therefore, early consideration of anti-HCV therapy is recommended in patients with HCV/HIV co-infection, given the risk of progressive liver disease. Indications for anti-HCV therapy in patients with HCV/HIV co-infection are generally similar to HCV mono-infection. Successful treatment of HCV reduces the risk of highly active antiretroviral therapy (HAART)-induced hepatotoxicity and improves the tolerability of these regimens, although SVR rates are lower compared to HIV-negative patients (Carrat et al., 2004).

Achievement of SVR significantly reduces overall mortality, liver-related mortality, and hepatic decompensation in patients co-infected with HCV and HIV (Berenguer et al., 2009). Correction of severe immunodeficiency (absolute CD4+ count <200 /μL) with HAART should be attempted prior to starting combination therapy for HCV. It may also be appropriate to delay anti-HCV therapy for several months after initiation of HAART so the initial adverse effects of two complicated regimens are not simultaneous. HAART has no direct anti-HCV effect and HCV-RNA levels usually remain unchanged (Matthews & Dore, 2008). Current guidelines acknowledge the lack of data on duration of anti-HCV therapy in patients with HIV co-infection and recommend an initial course of 48 weeks, regardless of HCV genotype. Following 48 weeks of therapy with PEG-IFN alfa-2a (180 μg weekly) and RBV (800 mg daily), 40% of patients with HCV/HIV co-infection achieve SVR (29% with genotype 1, 62% with genotypes 2 and 3). As in HIV-negative patients, early virologic response (EVR), defined by undetectable or 2 or greater log reduction of HCV-RNA levels by week 12 of treatment, is also an accurate predictor of SVR in HCV/HIV co-infection. Failure to achieve EVR in patients co-infected with HCV and HIV is reflected in an SVR of only 2% (Torriani et al., 2004).

HCV therapy in patients co-infected with HCV and HIV results in a higher frequency of side effects. For instance, RBV-induced hemolytic anemia occurs with higher frequency and is more severe in patients with HCV/HIV co-infection. This complication is of particular concern in patients treated with the nucleoside analogue zidovudine (AZT), which inhibits the hematopoietic response to RBV-induced hemolysis. The combination of RBV and didanosine (ddI), a nucleoside reverse transcriptase inhibitor, is contraindicated as it may result in severe mitochondrial toxicity leading to lactic acidosis, pancreatitis, myopathy, neuropathy, hepatic failure, and death (Ghany et al., 2009). A dose-dependent reduction of the white blood cell count and the absolute CD4+ count is anticipated with IFN but has not been implicated in the development of opportunistic infections (Ghany et al., 2009). Ritonavir, a protease inhibitor used to boost the effect of other protease inhibitors in HAART regimens, has important interactions with other antiviral agents, but no significant interactions have been reported when this drug is used concomitantly with PEG-IFN and RBV.

In conclusion, patients with HCV/HIV co-infection have worse outcomes compared to mono-infection with either virus. Although SVR rates are lower in co-infected patients, successful anti-HCV therapy is associated with better outcomes, including survival. PEG-IFN and RBV should be offered to good candidates for HCV therapy such as the patient described in the clinical vignette.

Treatment of Hepatitis C in Patients with Cirrhosis

Case: A 53-year-old Caucasian woman with biopsy-proven cirrhosis due to HCV genotype 1a infection is evaluated for antiviral therapy. The patient has compensated liver disease, as evidenced by a Child-Turcotte-Pugh score of 5 (class A) and has no other comorbidities that could be considered contraindications for antiviral therapy. White blood cell count and hemoglobin are normal but there is mild thrombocytopenia (120,000/μL). What is the role of anti-HCV therapy in patients with cirrhosis?

Extensive fibrosis is independently associated with diminished SVR in patients with HCV infection. For instance, SVR rates are lower (30% to 44%) with PEG-IFN and RBV in patients with bridging fibrosis or compensated cirrhosis due to HCV (predominantly genotype 1) (Manns et al., 2001). Combination therapy with PEG-IFN + RBV has been associated with histologic improvement in more than 50% of patients with bridging fibrosis or compensated cirrhosis, as well as a significant decrease in the incidence of clinical decompensation and HCC (Craxi, 2011). Patients with compensated cirrhosis, Child-Turcotte-Pugh (CTP) class A (Table 12.5), should be treated with PEG-IFN + RBV; however, close monitoring is required because of increased frequency of side effects.

The treatment of choice for decompensated cirrhosis is liver transplantation; however, only a minority of the pool of potential candidates benefit, and waiting times for liver transplantation continue to steadily increase as waiting lists grow. Combination therapy with PEG-IFN + RBV for 24 weeks in patients with decompensated cirrhosis (predominantly CTP class B) results in SVR rates of 44% (genotypes 2 and 3) and 7% (genotypes 1 and 4) (Iacobellis et al., 2007). In

Table 12.5 Child-Turcotte-Pugh Classification of Severity of Liver Disease		
Variable	**Points Scored**	
	1	**2**	**3**
Ascites	None	Easily controlled	Poorly controlled
Bilirubin (mg/dL)	<2	2–3	>3
INR	<1.7	1.7–2.3	>2.3
Albumin (g/dL)	>3.5	2.8–3.5	<2.8
Encephalopathy	None	Minimal	Severe
	Classification	
	A	**B**	**C**
Total points	5 or 6	7–9	10–15

one study, hepatic decompensation was 11 times less frequent over the subsequent 30 months in patients who achieved SVR compared to patients who did not achieve SVR and 17 times less frequent compared to untreated controls. Furthermore, 32% of untreated patients and 21% of patients who did not achieve SVR died during follow-up, compared to none of the patients who achieved SVR (Iacobellis et al., 2007). Successful anti-HCV therapy before liver transplantation in patients with decompensated cirrhosis has also been associated with a significant proportion of patients remaining HCV-RNA negative after transplantation (66% to 80%), therefore protecting the new graft against HCV infection (Everson et al., 2005; Forns et al., 2003). However, the safety of anti-HCV therapy in this population is a major concern because of the increased risk of profound bone marrow suppression, deteriorating hepatic function, and bacterial infections. Current guidelines acknowledge the benefits of IFN-based therapy in patients with decompensated cirrhosis (CTP class B and C) but also recognize that its efficacy is less well established by evidence, most of which is derived from a single randomized trial.

Cirrhotic patients who achieve an SVR remain at risk for HCC and other complications of their liver disease and require continued follow-up (Craxi, 2011).

Clinical trials evaluating the efficacy of the DAAs boceprevir and telaprevir have enrolled on average 20% to 30% of patients with advanced fibrosis/cirrhosis. These trials were not designed to assess the efficacy of DAAs in this particular subgroup, but improvements in SVR (approximately 50% and 30% to 70%, respectively) were noted when DAAs were added compared to standard therapy (Bacon et al., 2011; Jacobson et al., 2011; Poordad et al., 2011; Zeuzem et al., 2011). However, these data are derived from subgroup analyses and must be interpreted with caution until further research corroborates the effectiveness and safety of DAAs in patients with clinically overt cirrhosis.

In conclusion, anti-HCV therapy in patients with compensated and decompensated cirrhosis is associated with more frequent complications and should be administered only by experienced providers. Potential benefits include aborting the progression of liver disease and preventing allograft re-infection if the patient ultimately undergoes liver transplantation. The patient we describe is a candidate for therapy. The DAAs telaprevir and boceprevir have not been extensively studied in this population; therefore, no recommendations about their use can be made at this time.

Hepatitis C in Ethnic Minorities

Case: A 58-year-old Hispanic man with HCV genotype 1b infection is evaluated for antiviral treatment. Liver biopsy showed grade 3, stage 2 disease. The patient has no contraindications to antiviral therapy and agrees to start a combination of PEG-IFN alfa-2a and RBV. Is there any expected difference in SVR based on this patient's ethnicity compared to non-Hispanic White or African American individuals?

Epidemiologic data indicate that 3.2% of the African American population and 2.1% of the Hispanic population of the United States are anti-HCV seropositive, compared to 1.5% of non-Hispanic White (NHW) individuals (Alter et al., 1999). Despite the higher prevalence of HCV infection, Hispanic and African American populations have been generally underrepresented in therapeutic clinical trials evaluating anti-HCV regimens.

African American Population

HCV genotype 1 is by far the most common genotype in the United States (70%), with genotypes 2 and 3 representing most of the remaining 30%. However, the prevalence of genotype 1 infection is significantly higher in African Americans (97%) and SVR rates are lower compared to NHW patients infected with genotype 1 treated with PEG-IFN + RBV (21% to 28% vs. 37% to 52%, respectively) (Conjeevaram et al., 2006; Jacobson et al., 2007). Differences in SVR rates in African American patients compared to NHW populations are also evident with genotypes 2 and 3 infection (57% vs. 82%, respectively) (Shiffman et al., 2007). This unfavorable response may be explained by several viral and host-related factors. For instance, among viral factors, higher prevalence of genotype 1 infection and higher pretreatment HCV-RNA levels account for lower SVR rates. A novel host factor strongly associated with SVR in patients with HCV genotype 1 infection is the presence of single nucleotide polymorphisms near the gene coding for interferon-λ-3 or *IL28B*. The three *IL28B* genotypes are C/C, T/T, and T/C. The C/C genotype is associated with a favorable response to IFN therapy, whereas SVR is significantly lower in patients with either T/T or T/C genotypes. There are important differences in the prevalence of these genotypes among ethnic populations. For instance, there is a low prevalence of C/C genotype in African American compared to NHW populations (16% vs. 39%, respectively) (Ge et al., 2009). The CC genotype is associated with more than twofold greater SVR in African American individuals and therefore explains most of the unfavorable response to anti-HCV treatment in this group.

Data from recent trials studying DAAs show that African Americans treated with boceprevir or telaprevir in addition to standard therapy have a 20% to 45% greater SVR compared to standard therapy. However, even with DAA therapy, African Americans have approximately 15% lower SVR rates compared to NHW individuals ((Bacon et al., 2011; Jacobson et al., 2011; Poordad et al., 2011).

Hispanic Population

Hispanic patients also have lower SVR rates compared to NHW individuals across HCV genotypes. For instance, SVR is achieved in 34% of Hispanic versus 49% of NHW patients with genotype 1 infection treated with PEG-IFN alfa-2a and RBV (Rodriguez-Torres et al., 2009). Although infection with genotypes 2 and 3 is associated with higher SVR rates, the difference between Hispanic and NHW populations is also marked (66% vs. 87%, respectively) (Yu et al., 2009).

These unfavorable outcomes following antiviral therapy in Hispanic patients are independent of body mass index, sex, and HCV-RNA level. Furthermore, polymorphisms of the *IL28B* gene are also not wholly responsible for the differences in SVR because the frequency of the T/T or T/C genotypes is similar in Hispanic and NHW individuals (Ge et al., 2009). Data from subgroup analysis of a recent trial suggest that the addition of telaprevir to PEG-IFN + RBVn may abolish SVR differences among Hispanic and NHW populations (74% and 75%, respectively) (Jacobson et al., 2011).

In conclusion, Hispanic and African American individuals have had lower SVR rates compared to NHW individuals, regardless of HCV genotype (Table 12.6). Importantly, these differences persist in African Americans even with DAA therapy, which should be offered to the patient we describe in the vignette above.

Hepatitis C in Elderly Patients

Case: A 75-year-old Caucasian man with treatment-naïve HCV genotype 2a infection presents for anti-HCV therapy. A recent liver biopsy showed stage 3, grade 2 disease. Is the patient's age a contraindication for anti-HCV therapy?

Elderly patients have, in general, a lower prevalence of HCV infection compared to younger adults and children; however, as the population ages, an increase in the prevalence of this infection in elderly individuals is anticipated (Davis et al., 2010). Progression to fibrosis is accelerated when initial HCV infection occurs at older age, with the mean time from infection to cirrhosis halved compared to younger patients (16 vs. 33 years, respectively) (Minola et al., 2002).

Older age predicts a lower probability of being a candidate for anti-HCV treatment (Tsui et al., 2008). Furthermore, elderly patients are also more hesitant to accept treatment, and discontinuation and/or dosage reductions are more frequent in this age group compared to younger adults. The higher prevalence of comorbid conditions such as cardiovascular, renal, pulmonary, and hematologic diseases increases the risk of severe side effects and toxicity. Limited data suggest lower SVR rates in this population compared to younger adults (Floreani et al., 2006).

Table 12.6 Average Sustained Virologic Response Rates for HCV Genotypes in Different Ethnic Groups		
Ethnicity	**Average Sustained Virologic Response (%)**	
	Genotype 1	**Genotypes 2 and 3**
Non-Hispanic Whites	46	85
Hispanics	34	66
African Americans	24	57

Alter et al., 1999; Conjeevaram et al., 2006; Iacobellis et al., 2007; Jacobson et al., 2007; Shiffman et al., 2007.

In conclusion, as HCV-infected patients age, comorbidities unrelated to their liver disease will increase the complexity of antiviral therapy. Older age is not a contraindication to anti-HCV therapy, but careful selection of treatment candidates should be based on the patient's general health status. Data about the use of DAAs is also needed in this population.

References

Alter, M. J., D. Kruszon-Moran, O. V. Nainan, et al. (1999). Prevalence of hepatitis C virus infection in the United States, 1988 through 1994. *New England Journal of Medicine, 341*(8), 556–562.

Bacon, B. R., S. C. Gordon, E. Lawitz, et al. (2011). Boceprevir for previously treated chronic HCV genotype 1 infection. *New England Journal of Medicine, 364*(13), 1207–1217.

Berenguer, J., J. Alvarez-Pellicer, P. M. Mart'n, et al. (2009). Sustained virological response to interferon plus ribavirin reduces liver-related complications and mortality in patients coinfected with human immunodeficiency virus and hepatitis C virus. *Hepatology, 50*(2), 407–413.

Bonacini, M., H. J. Lin, & F. B. Hollinger (2001). Effect of coexisting HIV-1 infection on the diagnosis and evaluation of hepatitis C virus. *Journal of Acquired Immune Deficiency Syndrome, 26*(4), 340–344.

Carrat, F., F. Bani-Sadr, S. Pol, et al. (2004). Pegylated interferon alfa-2b vs standard interferon alfa-2b, plus ribavirin, for chronic hepatitis C in HIV-infected patients: a randomized controlled trial. *Journal of the American Medical Association, 292*(23), 2839–2848.

Carrion, J. A., M. Navasa, M. Garcia-Retortillo, et al. (2007). Efficacy of antiviral therapy on hepatitis C recurrence after liver transplantation: a randomized controlled study. *Gastroenterology, 132*(5), 1746–1756.

Conjeevaram, H. S., M. W. Fried, L. J. Jeffers, et al. (2006). Peginterferon and ribavirin treatment in African American and Caucasian American patients with hepatitis C genotype 1. *Gastroenterology, 131*(2), 470–477.

Craxi, A. (Feb. 28, 2011). EASL clinical practice guidelines: management of hepatitis C virus infection. *Journal of Hepatology* [Epub ahead of print].

Davis, G. L., M. J. Alter, H. El-Serag, T. Poynard, & L. W. Jennings (2010). Aging of hepatitis C virus (HCV)-infected persons in the United States: a multiple cohort model of HCV prevalence and disease progression. *Gastroenterology, 138*(2), 513–521.

Everson, G. T., J. Trotter, L. Forman, et al. (2005). Treatment of advanced hepatitis C with a low accelerating dosage regimen of antiviral therapy. *Hepatology, 42*(2), 255–262.

Fabrizi, F., F. F. Poordad, & P. Martin (2002). Hepatitis C infection and the patient with end-stage renal disease. *Hepatology, 36*(1), 3–10.

Fabrizi, F., P. Martin, V. Dixit, S. Bunnapradist, & G. Dulai (2004). Meta-analysis: Effect of hepatitis C virus infection on mortality in dialysis. *Alimentary Pharmacology & Therapeutics, 20*(11-12), 1271–1277.

Fabrizi, F., P. Martin, V. Dixit, S. Bunnapradist, & G. Dulai (2005). Hepatitis C virus antibody status and survival after renal transplantation: meta-analysis of observational studies. *American Journal of Transplantation, 5*(6), 1452–1461.

Fabrizi, F., V. Dixit, P. Messa, & P. Martin (2008). Interferon monotherapy of chronic hepatitis C in dialysis patients: meta-analysis of clinical trials. *Journal of Viral Hepatis, 15*(2), 79–88.

Floreani, A., E. Minola, I. Carderi, F. Ferrara, E. R. Rizzotto, & V. Baldo (2006). Are elderly patients poor candidates for pegylated interferon plus ribavirin in the treatment of chronic hepatitis C. *Journal of the American Geriatric Society, 54*(3), 549–550.

Forman, L. M., J. D. Lewis, J. A. Berlin, H. I. Feldman, & M. R. Lucey (2002). The association between hepatitis C infection and survival after orthotopic liver transplantation. *Gastroenterology, 122*(4), 889–896.

Forns, X., M. Garc´a-Retortillo, T. Serrano, et al. (2003). Antiviral therapy of patients with decompensated cirrhosis to prevent recurrence of hepatitis C after liver transplantation. *Journal of Hepatology, 39*(3), 389–396.

Ge, D., J. Fellay, A. J. Thompson, et al. (2009). Genetic variation in IL28B predicts hepatitis C treatment-induced viral clearance. *Nature, 461*(7262), 399–401.

Ghany, M. G., D. B. Strader, D. L. Thomas, & L. B. Seeff (2009). Diagnosis, management, and treatment of hepatitis C: an update. *Hepatology, 49*(4), 1335–1374.

Giordano, T. P., J. R. Kramer, J. Souchek, P. Richardson, & H. B. El-Serag (2004). Cirrhosis and hepatocellular carcinoma in HIV-infected veterans with and without the hepatitis C virus: a cohort study, 1992–2001. *Archives of Internal Medicine, 164*(21), 2349–2354.

Graham, C. S., L. R. Baden, E. Yu, et al. (2001). Influence of human immunodeficiency virus infection on the course of hepatitis C virus infection: a meta-analysis. *Clinical Infectious Diseases, 33*(4), 562–569.

Iacobellis, A., M. Siciliano, F. Perri, et al. (2007). Peginterferon alfa-2b and ribavirin in patients with hepatitis C virus and decompensated cirrhosis: a controlled study. *Journal of Hepatology, 46*(2), 206–212.

Jacobson, I. M., R. S. Brown Jr., J. McCone, et al. (2007). Impact of weight-based ribavirin with peginterferon alfa-2b in African Americans with hepatitis C virus genotype 1. *Hepatology, 46*(4), 982–990.

Jacobson, I. M., J. G. McHutchison, G. Dusheiko, et al. (2011). Telaprevir for previously untreated chronic hepatitis C virus infection. *New England Journal of Medicine, 364*(25), 2405–2416.

Kidney Disease: Improving Global Outcomes (2008). KDIGO clinical practice guidelines for the prevention, diagnosis, evaluation, and treatment of hepatitis C in chronic kidney disease. *Kidney International Supplement*, (109), S1–99.

Kim, J. H., G. Psevdos, J. Suh, & V. L. Sharp (2008). Co-infection of hepatitis B and hepatitis C virus in human immunodeficiency virus-infected patients in New York City, United States. *World Journal of Gastroenterology, 14*(43), 6689–6693.

Manns, M. P., J. G. McHutchison, S. C. Gordon, et al. (2001). Peginterferon alfa-2b plus ribavirin compared with interferon alfa-2b plus ribavirin for initial treatment of chronic hepatitis C: a randomised trial. *Lancet, 358*(9286), 958–965.

Matthews, G. V., & G. J. Dore. (2008). HIV and hepatitis C coinfection. *Journal of Gastroenterology & Hepatology, 23*(7 Pt 1), 1000–1008.

Minola, E., D. Prati, F. Suter, et al. (2001). Age at infection affects the long-term outcome of transfussion-associated chronic hepatitis C. *Blood, 99*(12), 4588–4591.

Poordad, F., J. McCone Jr., B. R. Bacon, et al. (2011). Boceprevir for untreated chronic HCV genotype 1 infection. *New England Journal of Medicine, 364*(13), 1195–1206.

Rendina, M., A. Schena, N. M. Castellaneta, et al. (2007). The treatment of chronic hepatitis C with peginterferon alfa-2a (40kDa) plus ribavirin in haemodialysed patients awaiting renal transplant. *Journal of Hepatology, 46*(5), 768–774.

Rodriguez-Torres, M., L. J. Jeffers, M. Y. Sheikh, et al. (2009). Peginterferon alfa-2a and ribavirin in Latino and non-Latino whites with hepatitis C. *New England Journal of Medicine, 360*(3), 257–267.

Rowe, I. A., K. Webb, B. K. Gunson, N. Mehta, S. Haque, & J. Neuberger (2008). The impact of disease recurrence on graft survival following liver transplantation: a single centre experience. *Transplant International, 21*(5), 459–465.

Shiffman, M. L., A. A. Mihas, F. Millwala, et al. (2007). Treatment of chronic hepatitis C virus in African Americans with genotypes 2 and 3. *American Journal of Gastroenterology, 102*(4), 761–766.

Spradling, P. R., J. T. Richardson, K. Buchacz, et al. (2010). Trends in hepatitis C virus infection among patients in the HIV outpatient study, 1996–2007. *Journal of Acquired Immune Deficiency Syndrome, 53*(3), 388–396.

Stravitz, R. T., M. L. Shiffman, A. J. Sanyal, et al. (2004). Effects of interferon treatment on liver histology and allograft rejection in patients with recurrent hepatitis C following liver transplantation. *Liver Transplantation, 10*(7), 850–858.

Thomas, D. L., J. Astemborski, R. M. Rai, et al. (2000). The natural history of hepatitis C virus infection: host, viral, and environmental factors. *Journal of the American Medical Association, 284*(4), 450–456.

Torriani, F. J., M. Rodriguez-Torres, J. K. Rockstroh, et al. (2004). Peginterferon Alfa-2a plus ribavirin for chronic hepatitis C virus infection in HIV-infected patients. *New England Journal of Medicine, 351*(5), 438–450.

Tsui, J. I., S. Currie, H. Shen, et al. (2008). Treatment eligibility and outcomes in elederly patients with chronic hepatitis C: results from the VA HCV-001 study. *Digestive Disease Science, 53*(3), 809–814.

Weber, R., C. A. Sabin, N. Friis-Moller, et al. (2006). Liver-related deaths in persons infected with the human immunodeficiency virus: the D:A:D study. *Archives of Internal Medicine, 166*(15), 1632–1641.

Yu, S., J. M. Douglass, C. Qualls, S. Arora, & J. C. Dunkelberg (2009). Response to therapy with pegylated interferon and ribavirin for chronic hepatitis C in Hispanics compared to non-Hispanic whites. *American Journal of Gastroenterology, 104*(7), 1686–1692.

Zeuzem, S., P. Andreone, S. Pol, et al. (2011). Telaprevir for retreatment of HCV infection. *New England Journal of Medicine, 364*(25), 2417–2428.

Chapter 13

New Treatments: Telaprevir and Boceprevir

Fred Poordad

Introduction

The hepatitis C virus (HCV) belongs to the Flaviviridae family, with a positive sense RNA genome that is single-stranded and 9,600 bases in length. Within both structural and nonstructural components of the genome, there are multiple potential targets for direct-acting antiviral agents (DAAs). The NS3/4A protease peptide leads to downstream cleavage of several other nonstructural proteins, and based on the experience with this class of agents in HIV therapy, it was a logical starting point for the development of HCV DAAs (Pawlotsky, 2007). This chapter focuses on the first two DAAs to gain FDA approval for HCV therapy, in conjunction with pegylated interferon (PEG-IFN) and ribavirin (RBV).

Telaprevir

Telaprevir (TVR) is an oral peptidomimetic NS3/4A inhibitor developed by Vertex Pharmaceuticals (Cambridge, MA). It is in the class of linear alpha keto-amide protease inhibitors and has antiviral activity primarily against genotype 1 hepatitis C virus. It may indeed have activity against other genotypes to a lesser extent but has not been formally evaluated in that respect.

Early-Phase Studies

The initial studies of TVR used monotherapy in healthy volunteers, followed by multiple ascending-dose studies over 3 days in HCV-infected patients. It showed robust antiviral activity, with a median viral decline of 4.77 $\log_{10}$ IU/mL with 750 mg every 8 hours, but only 3.49 $\log_{10}$ IU/mL with 1,250 mg every 12 hours, suggesting that thrice-daily dosing was the appropriate dosing schedule (Reesin, 2006). It was also clear from these early data that viral breakthrough was common with monotherapy, and that combination therapy would likely be necessary. This was further confirmed when a small pilot study compared TVR alone versus placebo or TVR with PEG-IFN for 14 days. The viral decline with combination therapy confirmed that PEG-IFN would need to be part of the treatment regimen (Forestier et al., 2007). Based on a combination study where patients were dosed with triple therapy for one month followed by PEG-IFN/ RBV for another 44 weeks, sustained virologic responses (SVRs) were achieved in some, leading to the phase 2 programs called PROVE (Protease Inhibition for Viral Evaluation).

Two programs, PROVE 1 and 2, were initiated in previously untreated HCV genotype 1 patients who were not cirrhotic or co-infected with HIV (Hezode et al., 2009; McHutchinson et al., 2009). SVR rates ranged from 35% to 67% across the arms, with the lowest SVR in the 12-week treatment arm (Fig. 13.1). A single arm in PROVE 2 lacked RBV, and this was instrumental in demonstrating the need for this agent. The rate of viral breakthrough was highest in that arm, suggesting that RBV decreases the resistance rates.

Another phase 2 study, PROVE 3, evaluated patients who had previously failed PEF-IFN + RBV (McHutchinson et al., 2010). In this study, 24 weeks of TVR was evaluated with 48 weeks of PEG-IFN + RBV, compared to the 12 weeks of TVR with 24 weeks of PEG-IFN + RBV. While there was no difference in efficacy, there was a higher discontinuation rate due to adverse events in the longer treatment arm, suggesting that TVR dosing beyond week 12 was not feasible (Fig. 13.2).

Phase III Data

ADVANCE and ILLUMINATE

Two large phase 3 trials assessed treatment-naïve patients. The ADVANCE (A New Direction in HCV Care: A Study of Treatment-Naïve Hepatitis C Patients with Telaprevir) trial was a multicenter, multinational study of 1,088 patients, of whom 21% had advanced fibrosis. Although there was an 8- and 12-week treatment duration arm of TVR 750 mg orally every 8 hours compared to a control of 48 weeks of PEG-IFN + RBV, the 12-week duration appeared to have higher sustained response rates (Fig. 13.3) (Jacobson et al., 2011).

A response-guided treatment (RGT) paradigm was used whereby patients who became undetectable by week 4 and remained so until week 12 (extended rapid virologic response [eRVR]) were treated with only 24 weeks of PEG-IFN + RBV (T12PR24), compared to those who responded more slowly

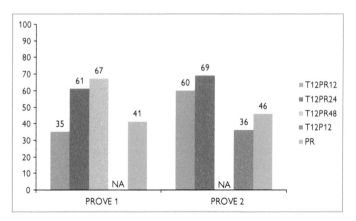

Figure 13.1 PROVE 1 and 2 SVR rates. T, telaprevir; P, pegylated interferon; R, ribavirin; numbers denote duration of therapy for each medication in weeks. NA, arm did not exist for that study.

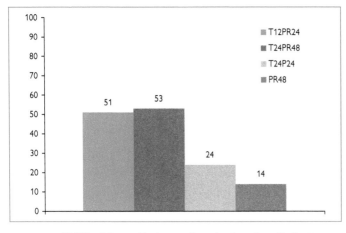

Figure 13.2 PROVE 3 SVR rates. T, telaprevir; P, pegylated interferon; R, ribavirin; numbers denote duration of therapy for each medication in weeks.)

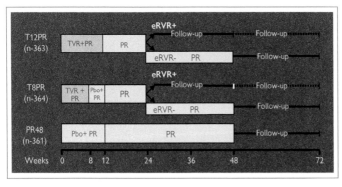

Figure 13.3 Design of the ADVANCE trial. T or TVR, telaprevir 750 mg q8h. Pbo, placebo. P, PEG-IFN alfa-2a 180 µg/wk. R, ribavirin 1,000 or 1,200 mg/day. Roche TaqMan® v2 LLOQ of 25 IU/mL.

and required 48 weeks of PEG-IFN + RBV (T12PR48). This shortened therapy benefited 58% of patients (Fig. 13.4). The overall SVR rates were 75% for the T12PR arm, 69% for T8PR, and 44% for control, both experimental arms being superior to control. In those with eRVR in the T12PR arm, 89% achieved SVR, whereas those without eRVR in the same arm had SVR rates of 54%. Adverse events led to all treatment discontinuation in 10% of the T12PR arm versus 7% in the control group, whereas the study drug alone was discontinued in 11% during the first 12 weeks in the T12PR arm versus only 1% in the control arm.

The most notable adverse events in the phase 3 trials are listed in Table 13.1. Although rash was common, occurring in more than half of the patients, severe rash, defined as involving more than 50% of the body surface area, occurred in fewer than 10%, with study drug discontinuation in 7% in the

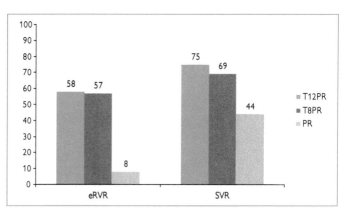

Figure 13.4 ADVANCE eRVR and SVR rates. T, telaprevir; P, pegylated interferon; R, ribavirin; numbers denote duration of therapy for each medication in weeks.

Table 13.1 Telaprevir: Most Notable Adverse Events in Phase 3 Trials		
Adverse Event ≥5% Frequency	Telaprevir-Containing Regimen	PEG-IFN + RBV Control
Uric acid elevation	73	29
Bilirubin elevation	41	28
Rash	56	34
Fatigue	56	50
Nausea	39	28
Anemia	36	17
Diarrhea	26	17
Vomiting	13	8
Hemorrhoids	12	3
Anorectal discomfort	11	3
Dysgeusia	10	3
Anal pruritus	6	1

T12PR arm versus 1% in PEG-IFN + RBV control. The more novel adverse event noted in the study was that of anorectal disorders, which occurred at a rate of close to 30% and included anal burning, pruritus, and hemorrhoids. These symptoms rarely led to study drug discontinuation. Anemia (hemoglobin <10 g/dL) occurred in 38% of patients (14% in PEG-IFN + RBV control), and severe anemia (<8.5 g/dL) was noted in 9% of TVR patients compared to 2% of controls.

A companion study called ILLUMINATE (Illustrating the Effects of Combination Therapy with Telaprevir) was conducted in open-label fashion without control to assess if patients demonstrating eRVR could indeed be treated with 24 weeks of PEG-IFN + RBV compared to 48 weeks (Sherman et al., 2011). Patients were randomized based on eRVR status at week 20 to receive either 24 or 48 weeks of PEG-IFN + RBV. The overall SVR was 72%, with no difference in those with eRVR receiving 24 versus 48 weeks of PEG-IFN + RBV, with SVR rates of 92% and 88%, respectively (Fig. 13.5). Study discontinuation in this open-label study of all study drugs occurred in 17% of patients, but adverse events were very similar to the ADVANCE trial.

These two trials demonstrated the superiority of a TVR-based regimen over control and the sound strategy of using RGT to shorten therapy in patients achieving eRVR. The notable adverse events of rash, anemia, and anorectal discomfort could be managed in the majority of patients, with relatively few TVR discontinuations.

REALIZE

The REALIZE (Re-treatment of Patients with Telaprevir-Based Regimen to Optimize Outcomes) trial was the name of the registration phase 3 trial for the previous PEG-IFN + RBV treatment failure population (Zeuzem et al., 2011). Based on the findings of the PROVE 3 trial, it was determined that 48 weeks of PEG-IFN + RBV with 12 weeks of TVR would be the paradigm for all patients in the phase 3 trial. Hence, all arms of REALIZE trial were 48 weeks in duration (Fig. 13.6). One of the arms had the experimental 4-week lead-in (LI) of PEG-IFN + RBV preceding 12 weeks of triple therapy, followed by 32 weeks of PEG/RBV. The SVR rates of the three arms were 66% in the LI arm, 64% in the T12PR48 arm, and 17% in the control arm (Fig. 13.7). In a pooled analysis of both study arms, relapsers had the highest SVR at 86% (24% control), followed by those who had a partial response to previous treatment at 57% (15% control), and finally, null responders at 31% (5% control).

FDA Label

The label issued by the FDA for TVR is for chronic hepatitis C, genotype 1 patients, regardless of past treatment history. The key differences in the label issued and the clinical trials is that previous PEG-IFN + RBV relapse patients were studied in the REALIZE trial with a 48-week backbone of PEG-IFN + RBV

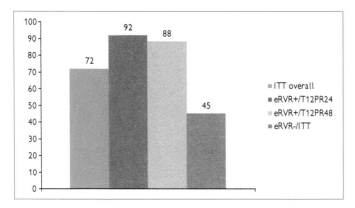

Figure 13.5 ILLUMINATE SVR rates. T, telaprevir; P, pegylated interferon; R, ribavirin; numbers denote duration of therapy for each medication in weeks. ITT, intention to treat.

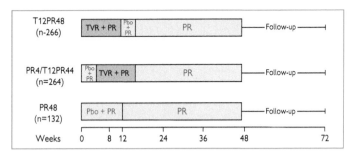

Figure 13.6 Design of the REALIZE trial. T or TVR, telaprevir 750 mg q8h, Pbo, Placebo. P, PEG-IFN alfa-2a 180 µg/wk. R, ribavirin 1,000 or 1,200 mg/day. Roche TaqMan® v2 LLOQ of 25 IU/mL.

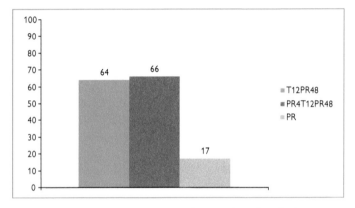

Figure 13.7 REALIZE SVR rates. T, telaprevir; P, pegylated interferon; R, ribavirin; numbers denote duration of therapy for each medication in weeks.

but are eligible per the label for RGT in the same way that treatment-naïve patients are. Another difference between the label and the clinical trials are the stopping rules, which suggest all three drugs be discontinued if at weeks 4 or 12 there is a viral load of greater than 1,000 IU/mL (Table 13.2). Additionally, the overall SVR rate in the ADVANCE trial in the T12PR arm was modified to 79% while the control arm was increased to 46% after changing some of values that were below the limits of quantification, but detectable, with the rationale that these were likely false-positive values.

Boceprevir

Boceprevir (BOC; Merck and Co., Whitehouse Station, NJ) is a peptidomimetic ketoamide NS3 protease inhibitor that forms a covalent, reversible bond at the active site. It is predominantly active against genotype 1, but in a small

Table 13.2 Stopping Rules for Telaprevir			
Regimen	Time	Criterion	Action
TVR+PEG-IFN/RBV	Week 4 or week 12	HCV RNA >1,000 IU/mL	Discontinue all therapy
	Week 24	Detectable HCV RNA	Discontinue PR

series was almost as active against genotype 3 (Silva et al., 2011). It has not been rigorously evaluated for any genotype other than 1, however.

Early-Phase Studies

A 14-day phase 1 monotherapy study evaluating 100 to 400 mg of BOC revealed an RNA decline of 2.06 $\log_{10}$ using 400 mg, but with viral breakthrough occurring in several patients (Sarrazin et al., 2007). The addition of PEG-IFN alfa-2b in a randomized, double-blind crossover study evaluated patients who did not achieve a 2 log decline at 12 weeks using PEG/RBV (null responders). BOC monotherapy (200 to 400 mg TID) for one week was followed by either PEG-IFN alfa-2b (1.5 mg/kg) weekly for 2 weeks or combination PEG-IFN alfa-2b plus BOC for 2 weeks. With combination therapy using PEG-IFN and 400 mg BOC, the mean reduction in HCV RNA was 2.68 $\log_{10}$, significantly higher than with monotherapy using either compound alone. There were no observed differences in safety parameters, but 400 mg was the maximum dose tested in phase 1 studies.

The initial phase 2 program (RESPOND 1) again selected a null responder population to test various BOC doses with and without RBV (Schiff et al., 2008). A total of 357 null responders to PEG-IFN/RBV were enrolled in several arms assessing 100/200/400/800 mg of BOC TID with PEG-IFN-2b/RBV (Fig. 13.8), None of the arms initially had triple therapy with 800 mg BOC and PEG-IFN-2b/RBV, but after an interim analysis by the Data Safety Monitoring Board, a protocol amendment placed all patients demonstrating viral reductions below 10,000 IU/mL on this regimen. Given the high rate of resistance that developed due to the inadequate initial dosing, the overall SVR rates were 14% or lower. Based on this study, it was determined that the null responder population may not be well suited to triple therapy. It was also determined that RBV was likely necessary, and patients who showed IFN responsiveness were ultimately the ones who had a likelihood of achieving SVR with the addition of BOC.

The treatment-naïve phase 2 trial, called SPRINT 1 (Serine Protease Inhibitor Therapy 1), was a multicenter, multinational study with several arms assessing 800 mg TID of BOC with PEG-IFN-2b/RBV (Kwo et al., 2010) (Fig. 13.9). Varying durations of 24 to 48 weeks were assessed, with an assessment of a LI concept of 4 weeks of PEG-IFN-2b/RBV prior to starting BOC. A single arm using a lower RBV dose was also assessed.

The LI rationale was initially based on pharmacokinetic parameters of achieving steady-state trough levels of both IFN and RBV, thereby potentially decreasing the likelihood of developing viral breakthrough and resistance when BOC was added. In this study of 595 patients, with roughly 100 patients in each arm, up to 17% were black, and up to 9% had cirrhosis. The highest SVR achieved was 75% in the arm that had a 4-week LI, followed by 44 weeks of triple therapy (Fig. 13.10). In both LI arms, the SVR

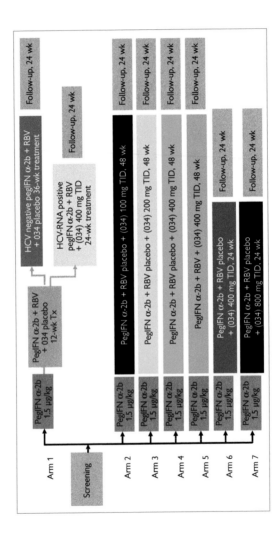

Figure 13.8 RESPOND 1 trial design.

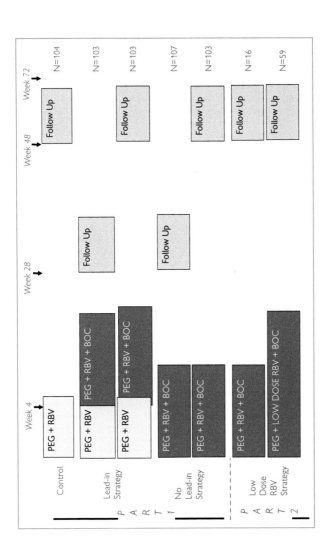

Figure 13.9 SPRINT 1 trial design.

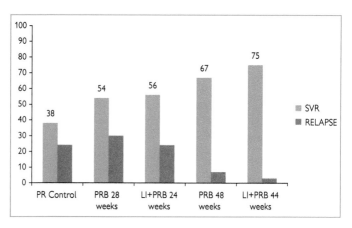

Figure 13.10 SPRINT 1 SVR and relapse rates (part 1 of study).

rates were slightly higher than the corresponding arms without LI, though not powered to show a difference in efficacy. The viral decline during the LI phase predicted the likelihood of achieving SVR (Fig. 13.11). A small difference in viral breakthrough was also noted in the LI arms. Based on this, the LI concept was subsequently adopted for future studies. All BOC-containing arms were significantly higher than control, including the black patient population, with a maximum 53% SVR compared to historical controls. The most common treatment-emergent adverse events were anemia, nausea, vomiting, and dysgeusia. Erythropoietin-stimulating agents (ESAs) were allowed in the study at the discretion of the investigators for patients developing hemoglobin declines below 10 g/dL. Both anemia and the use of ESAs (used in the majority of anemic patients) were noted to be associated with increased SVR. This led to an exploratory study assessing ESA versus RBV dose reduction, with results expected in 2012.

Phase 3 Trials

A 1,097-patient study of treatment-naïve patients called SPRINT 2 enrolled two cohorts of patients, one non-black and one black (Poordad et al., 2011). The intent was to study the black population independently to more clearly characterize this historically less responsive population. The control arm was 48 weeks of PEG-2b/RBV with the main experimental arm being a 4-week LI, followed by 44 weeks of PEG-2b/RBV with BOC 800 mg TID (Fig. 13.12). An exploratory RGT arm allowed a shortened duration of therapy of 28 weeks for patients who became HCV RNA undetectable below 9.3 IU/mL by treatment week 8 and remained negative to week 24. Patients who became undetectable after week 8 but by week 24 received 4 weeks of LI, 24 weeks of triple therapy, and then a "tail" of 20 weeks of PEG/RBV. The overall SVR rates were 63%

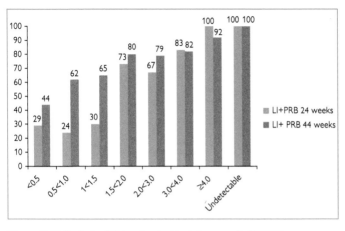

Figure 13.11 Predicting SVR based on lead-in viral response in SPRINT 1.

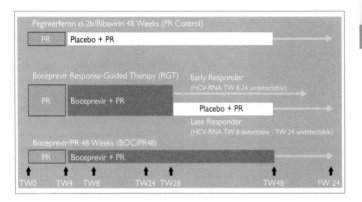

Figure 13.12 SPRINT 2 trial design.

(68% in non-black patients and 53% in blacks vs. 40% and 23%, respectively, in controls; $p = 0.004$ and $p = 0.044$) (Fig. 13.13). A total of 57% of patients were eligible for short-duration therapy based on becoming undetectable by week 8. The SVR in this cohort who completed therapy was 96% in both the RGT arm and the 4+44-week arm, suggesting that the duration of therapy could be shortened for rapid responders. The predominant adverse events were anemia and dysgeusia. Anemia occurred in almost 50% of patients, the majority of whom received ESA with RBV dose reduction, which was more common in the BOC arms.

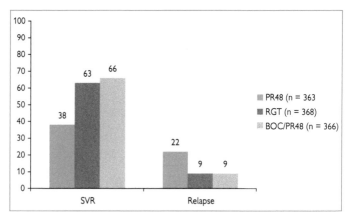

Figure 13.13 SPRINT 2 SVR and relapse rates.

The corresponding treatment-experienced study, called RESPOND 2 (Retreatment with HCV Serine Protease Inhibitor Boceprevir and Peginteron/Rebetol-2), assessed 403 patients who were either previous partially IFN-responsive nonresponders or relapsers, and excluded null responder patients (Bacon et al., 2011) (Fig. 13.14). The SVR rates were 66% in the 48-week arm and 59% in the RGT arm, both of which were significantly better than control (21%; $p < 0.0001$) (Fig. 13.15). The LI paradigm was used in this study as well, and almost one quarter of patients demonstrated less than a 1 $\log_{10}$ decline in HCV RNA at the end of LI, suggesting poor IFN response. These patients had SVR rates of 34%; those who demonstrated more than a 1 $\log_{10}$ decline in HCV RNA during LI had SVR rates of 73% to 79%, with correspondingly lower rates of resistant variants as well. Anemia rates of 50% were seen, but only 2% of patients discontinued treatment for this adverse event.

FDA Label

The FDA label issued for BOC differs in some respects from the clinical trials. The treatment-naïve patients, partial responders, and relapsers are all eligible for shorter-duration therapy if virus is undetectable by treatment week 8. This would be a LI plus 24 weeks of triple therapy for naïve patients, and a LI plus 32 weeks for the other groups. These same patients would all receive a LI plus 32 weeks of triple therapy followed by 12 more weeks of just PEG-IFN and RBV if they are not undetectable by week 8 but are less than 100 IU/mL by week 12. For those with viral levels above 100 IU/mL by week 12, or with any detectable virus at week 24, all three drugs are discontinued. Although 12-week null responder patients were not studied in the RESPOND 2 trial, the FDA granted a label for a LI followed by 44 weeks of triple therapy, the same regimen recommended for all cirrhotic patients.

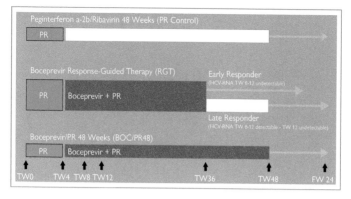

Figure 13.14 RESPOND 2 trial design.

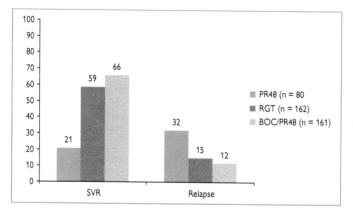

Figure 13.15 RESPOND 2 SVR and relapse rates.

Conclusion

Both of these new DAAs, telaprevir and boceprevir, are major advances in the treatment of hepatitis C. The SVR rates are nearly double what they were previously, and the paradigm of RGT applies to a substantial number of patients, shortening the course of therapy to less than 48 weeks. Due to the adverse event profiles, the TID dosing regimen, and the reliance on IFN, other therapies will eventually supplant these two compounds. However, their place in history as the first compounds to usher in a new treatment era is secure.

References

Bacon, B. R., S. C. Gordon, E. Lawitz, et al. (2011). Boceprevir for treatment of chronic hepatitis C genotype 1 nonresponders. *New England Journal of Medicine, 364,* 1207–1217.

Forestier, N., et al. (2007). Antiviral activity of telaprevir (VX-950) and peginterferon alfa-2a in patients with hepatitis C. *Hepatology, 46,* 640–647.

Hezode, C., et al. (2009). Telaprevir and peginterferon with or without ribavirin for chronic HCV infection. *New England Journal of Medicine, 360*(18), 1839–1850.

Jacobson, I. M., J. G. McHutchison, G. Dusheiko, et al.; ADVANCE Study Team (2011). Telaprevir for previously untreated chronic hepatitis C virus infection. *New England Journal of Medicine, 364*(25), 2405–2416.

Kwo, P. Y., et al. (2010). Efficacy of boceprevir, an NS3 protease inhibitor, in combination with peginterferon alfa-2b and ribavirin in treatment-naive patients with genotype 1 hepatitis C infection (SPRINT-1): an open-label, randomised, multicentre phase 2 trial. *Lancet, 376*(9742), 705–716.

McHutchinson, J. G., et al. (2009). Telaprevir with peginterferon and ribavirin for chronic HCV genotype 1 infection. *New England Journal of Medicine, 360*(18), 1827–1838.

McHutchinson, J. G., et al. (2010). Telaprevir for previously treated chronic HCV infection. *New England Journal of Medicine, 362*(14), 1292–1303.

Pawlotsky, J. M. (2007). The hepatitis C viral life cycle as a target for new antiviral therapies. *Gastroenterology, 132,* 1979–1998.

Poordad, F., J. McCone, B. Bacon, et al., for the SPRINT 2 Investigators. (2011). Boceprevir with peginterferon and ribavirin for chronic hepatitis C. *New England Journal of Medicine, 364,* 1195–1206.

Reesink, H. W. (2006). Rapid decline of viral RNA in hepatitis C patients treated with VX-950: a phase 1b, placebo-controlled, randomized study. *Gastroenterology. 131,* 997–1002.

Sarrazin, C., et al. (2007). SCH 503034, a novel hepatitis C virus protease inhibitor, plus pegylated interferon alpha-2b for genotype 1 nonresponders. *Gastroenterology, 132*(4), 1270–1278.

Schiff, E., et al. (2008). Boceprevir (B) combination therapy in null responders (NR): Response dependent on interferon responsiveness. *Journal of Hepatology, 48,* S46.

Sherman, K. E., S. L. Flamm, N. H. Afdhal, et al.; ILLUMINATE Study Team (2011). Response-guided telaprevir combination treatment for hepatitis C virus infection. *New England Journal of Medicine, 365*(11), 1014–1024.

Silva, M., C. Kasserra, S. Gupta, et al. (2011). Antiviral activity of boceprevir monotherapy in treatment-naïve subjects with chronic hepatitis C genotype 2/3. *Hepatology International, 5,* 259.

Zeuzem, S., P. Andreone, S. Pol, et al.; REALIZE Study Team (2011). Telaprevir for retreatment of HCV infection. *New England Journal of Medicine, 364*(25), 2417–2428.

Chapter 14

HCV Directly Acting Antiviral Therapies (Other than Boceprevir and Telaprevir)

Joseph Ahn and Steven L. Flamm

Introduction

Hepatitis C virus (HCV) affects approximately 170 million people worldwide and is a leading cause of chronic liver disease in the United States. It is the most common indication for liver transplantation (Armstrong et al., 2006). Treatment with pegylated interferon-alfa (PEG) and ribavirin (RBV) has been the standard of care for many years; unfortunately, sustained virologic response (SVR) rates of only 40% to 45% in patients with HCV genotype 1, the most common genotype in the United States, are achieved (Fried et al., 2002; Manns et al., 2001). The relatively poor response rates in genotype 1 patients have provided the impetus for investigation of improved therapies for HCV. Many compounds are under study. The most advanced area of research is in the class of antiviral therapy known as the directly acting antiviral (DAA) therapies. Unlike PEG and RBV, these compounds target specific steps in the HCV life cycle, especially those involving post-translation processing and replication.

Boceprevir and telaprevir, both NS3/4A protease inhibitors (PIs), have been recently approved by the FDA for treatment of HCV patients with genotype 1. Although their approval represents a milestone in the treatment of HCV, significant limitations remain. First, the antiviral regimen is poorly tolerated. In fact, many patients have contraindications to PEG and RBV and are ineligible to receive these medications. Second, there are numerous drug–drug interactions that may limit the usage of the first generation of PIs. Third, the medications are administered thrice daily with food. This will likely represent a problem for medication adherence. Fourth, the issue of resistance-associated variants (RAVs) is important with DAAs. The PIs are highly potent; however, HCV is an RNA virus and is characterized by a high mutation rate. RAVs may exist prior to antiviral therapy or may develop on therapy. Thus, these medications cannot be administered as monotherapy or without both PEG and RBV (Hezode et al., 2009). The significance of RAVs is as of yet poorly understood; although the majority of mutant variants are replaced by wild-type virus within 3 to 7 months of boceprevir and telaprevir discontinuation, these mutants may be detectable for up to several years after treatment discontinuation. This potential for emergence of drug resistance must be considered a major threat because of the risk of broader cross-resistance to other compounds in the NS3/4A PI class, which may significantly reduce future treatment options. Fifth, these medications are indicated only for patients with HCV genotype 1. There are patients with HCV genotype 2 or 3 who have failed PEG and RBV therapy and require a therapeutic alternative. HCV genotype 4 has not yet been investigated with telaprevir or boceprevir. This group of patients also requires more effective regimens. Finally, SVR rates with telaprevir or boceprevir in challenging patient populations such as those with previous treatment failure, significant hepatic fibrosis, HIV/HCV co-infection, or of African American descent are not as robust as in the general population or have not yet been well studied. All of these issues indicate that there will be many patients who are not served by the first generation of PIs. Thus, there remains interest in the pursuit of alternative DAAs that target other steps in the HCV life cycle, such as the NS5B polymerase, NS5A protein, and NS4B protein.

Newer DAAs must address limitations with the current NS3/4A, PEG, and RBV regimen. An optimal DAA should be more potent, result in decreased treatment duration and increased SVR, be administered once or twice daily preferably without food intake, and be pan-genotypic. Ideally, the next generation of compounds would be well tolerated and offer a complementary mechanism of action to DAAs in other classes so that interferon-free regimens would be possible.

The purpose of this chapter is to review other DAAs in development that may, in the near future, represent an advance in the antiviral regimen for HCV as we look beyond the recently approved first-generation NS3/4A PIs. The focus will be on therapies that have progressed into phase 2 trials. It should be noted that the reports on these therapies are preliminary and are often in abstract form.

HCV Physiology

To understand the potential new targets of DAA therapy, the physiology of HCV protein synthesis will be reviewed. Although the precise mechanisms of HCV replication are incompletely understood, especially with regard to replication-complex assembly and RNA synthesis, due to limited in vitro models of HCV replication, there have been advances in understanding in recent years (Sklan et al., 2009). The main steps of the HCV life cycle include entry into the host cell, viral uncoating, translation of structural and nonstructural HCV proteins, replication, assembly of the viral proteins, and subsequent virus release (Fig. 14.1). Potential targets for DAAs exist at each step of this replication cycle.

Host cell surface molecules such as CD81 and human scavenger receptor class B type I (SR-BI) that interact with HCV to facilitate cell viral entry have been identified as possible inhibition targets. Once inside the hepatocyte, HCV undergoes uncoating and viral genome translation into a large polyprotein. The

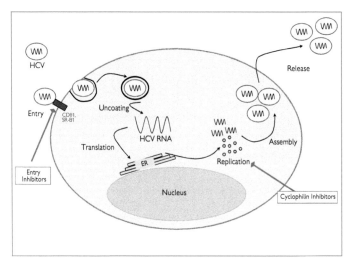

Figure 14.1 The HCV life cycle begins with entry into the host cell through recognition of host surface molecules such as CD81 and SR-B1. Viral uncoating leads to exposure of the viral genome, which in turns undergoes translation using the host cell machinery into structural and nonstructural HCV proteins, which are critical in proceeding with viral replication and assembly into new HCV particles. Finally, these new HCV viruses are released into the host. Potential host-targeted antiviral agents include entry inhibitors and cyclophilin inhibitors.

polyprotein is processed by host and viral proteases to form at least ten non-structural or structural protein products. Structural proteins include the virus core, and envelope proteins E1 and E2. Nonstructural proteins include P7, NS2, NS3, NS4A, NS4B, NS5A, and NS5B (Fig. 14.2). The nonstructural proteins are vital for viral replication and assembly of new HCV virions. After processing of the polyprotein, the nonstructural proteins establish the machinery for viral replication in close association with intracellular membranes. NS2 is an autoprotease that is essential for completion of the HCV replication cycle, although its exact function has yet to be delineated. The NS3 protease is critical in cleaving the large polyprotein into its various components and also has a role in inactivating host proteins that modulate interferon-mediated innate immunity. NS4A is an anchoring peptide that anchors the NS3 protein to the cellular membrane and acts as a cofactor for the NS3 protease. NS4B is thought to induce the formation of a replication complex, known as the membranous web, to act as the platform for replication. The role of the NS5A protein in the HCV life cycle is not well understood, although it is associated with the replication complex. Cyclophilins are a highly conserved family of human enzymes (peptidyl-prolyl cis-trans isomerases) involved in protein folding, transport, and secretion, mitochondrial function, and immune response. Cyclophilins can be co-opted by the hepatitis C virus to become a cofactor for viral replication. In

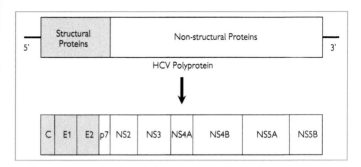

Figure 14.2 The polyprotein is processed by host and viral proteases to form non-structural or structural protein products. Structural proteins include the virus core (C), and envelope proteins E1 and E2. Nonstructural proteins include P7, NS2, NS3, NS4A, NS4B, NS5A, and NS5B.

hepatocytes, cyclophilins A and B bind with NS5A and NS5B to help form a replication complex to mediate the correct folding and trafficking of HCV proteins, thus functioning as a positive modulator for hepatitis C viral replication (Liu et al., 2009; Watashi et al., 2005). The NS5B is an RNA-dependent RNA polymerase that synthesizes HCV RNA. Subsequently, the virions are assembled and released (Cheng et al., 2011).

NS3/4A PIs

NS3/4A PIs are effective via inhibitory competition and have genotype activity specific against genotype 1 (1b > 1a). Telaprevir and boceprevir are members of this class. PIs have a low resistance barrier and have a high risk of cross-resistance within the class.

Danoprevir (RG-7227/ITMN-191) is a potent, non-covalent, macrocyclic PI that selectively blocks the NS3/4A protease (Forestier et al., 2011). In combination with PEG and RBV, danoprevir was reported to yield undetectable HCV RNA rates of 88% to 92% at week 12 compared to 43% in the control PEG/RBV group in 225 HCV genotype 1, treatment-naïve, noncirrhotic subjects (Terrault et al., 2010). Using ritonavir boosting, taking advantage of the cytochrome p450 metabolism of the drug, BID dosing was shown to be safe and robust in a recent study (Rouzier et al., 2011). More importantly, danoprevir was used in a PEG/RBV-sparing DAA combination regimen with mericitabine, an NS5B nucleoside inhibitor, in the INFORM study, which will be discussed later in this chapter.

BMS-650032, another NS3 PI, was studied in combination with PEG/RBV in 47 noncirrhotic, genotype 1, treatment-naïve patients. This phase 2a study compared 3 doses (200 mg BID, 600 mg BID, 600 mg qd) of BMS-650032 against placebo for a total of 48 weeks. The extended rapid virologic response (eRVR), defined as undetectable HCV RNA (<10 IU/mL) at weeks 4 and 12 of treatment, was the main endpoint. The eRVR rate was 75% to 91.7% in the BMS-

650032 arms, compared to 0% (0/11) in the placebo + PEG/RBV control arm. Adverse events were similar to those associated with PEG/RBV, although ALT elevations were more frequently noted in the BMS-650032 arms compared to control (Bronowicki et al, 2011). The results of combination therapy with BMS-650032 and BMS-790052, an NS5A replication complex inhibitor, will be discussed later.

BI-201335 is a non-covalent, linear NS3/4A PI that has a half-life of approximately 20 to 30 hours, supporting daily dosing. It also has marginal cytochrome p450 metabolism, reducing the risk for drug–drug interactions. BI-201335 was shown to be potent, leading to a 4.4 log 10 HCV RNA decline in 15 days of monotherapy at 240 mg qd (Manns et al., 2011). However, two trials using BI-201335 with PEG/RBV in treatment-naïve (SILEN-C1) and treatment-experienced (SILEN-C2) HCV genotype 1 patients reported development of jaundice in nearly 30% and rash in 20% to 30%. SILEN-C1 reported an SVR of 83% in the combination BI-201335/PEG/RBV without a PEG/RBV lead-in (3 days) compared to 73% with the lead-in at the 240-mg BI-201335 dose (Sulkowski et al., 2011a). In SILEN-C2, an SVR of 47% was reported with the 240-mg daily dose (Sulkowski et al., 2011b). Although indirect hyperbilirubinemia, especially in those with Gilbert's syndrome, was not uncommon, the potential of the drug, based on its potency and improved dosing and drug interaction profile, led to the continuation of its study in a phase 3 study.

TMC-435 is a non-covalent, macrocyclic NS3/4A PI that offers daily dosing (Reesink et al., 2010). The PILLAR study reported on 386 HCV genotype I, treatment-naïve patients who were treated with TMC-435 and combination PEG/RBV. At week 4, 68% to 79% of patients had undetectable virus. At week 12, 91% to 97% were undetectable. This compares to 5% (week 4) and 58% (week 12), respectively, in the PEG/RBV control group. There were no significant adverse events reported (Fried et al., 2010). The ASPIRE trial was a phase 2b study that enrolled 396 HCV genotype 1, treatment-experienced patients. Patients received TMC-435 with PEG/RBV or PEG/RBV control. At week 24, 69% to 93% of the triple therapy patients had undetectable virus compared to 52% in the control group. As expected, SVR was superior in relapsers compared to null responders (Zeuzem et al., 2011).

Vaniprevir (MK-7009) is a non-covalent, macrocyclic NS3/4A PI that was shown in a phase 2a study of 94 genotype 1 treatment-naïve patients to be effective in combination with PEG/RBV. The rapid virologic response (RVR) rate was 67% to 84% in the vaniprevir arms versus 5% in the PEG/RBV control arm. SVR was reported to be 78% to 84% in the vaniprevir/PEG/RBV arms compared with 63% in the control arm (Manns et al., 2010).

ACH-1625 is an open-chain, non-covalent, NS3 PI that was shown to have high antiviral potency, high liver/plasma concentration ratios, and no serious adverse events in a phase 2a trial. It produced a 75% to 81% RVR after 5 days of treatment in both treatment-naïve and -experienced, HCV genotype 1 patients (Detishin et al., 2011). Segment 2 of the phase 2 trial was initiated based upon these promising findings.

ABT-450 is an NS3/4a PI that was boosted with ritonavir and studied in 35 HCV genotype 1 treatment-naïve patients with a 3-day monotherapy lead-in followed by 12 weeks of ABT-450/ritonavir with PEG/RBV, followed by PEG/RBV through week 48. 88% of the ABT-450 group had RVR compared with 9% in the placebo arm. 92% had undetectable HCV RNA at 12 weeks, with no virologic rebound. Ritonavir-boosted ABT-450 groups had similar adverse events and tolerance compared to the control groups. Side effects were consistent with those attributed to PEG/RBV (Lawitz et al., 2011a). Studies with the NS3/4A PIs under development are reviewed in Table 14.1.

Table 14.1 DAAs In Development		
NS3/4A PIs	**Non-nucleoside NS5B PIs**	**Nucleos(t)ide NS5B PIs**
ABT-450	ABT-072	Mericitabine (RG-7128)
ACH-1625	ABT-333	MK-0608
BI-201335	ANA-598	PSI-7977
BMS-791325	BI-1941	PSI-938
Danoprevir (RG-7227/ ITMN-191)	BI-207127	RG-7348
GS-9256	Filibuvir (PF-00868554)	TMC-649128
GS-9451	GS-9190	*IDX-184*
MK-5172	IDX-375	*R-1626*
PHX-1766	Tegobuvir (GS-9190)	*Valopicitabine (NM-283)*
TMC-435	VX-222	
Vaniprevir (MK-7009)	VX-759	**NS5A Inhibitors**
VX-985	VX-916	ABT-267
Ciluprevir (BILN-2061)	*BILB 1941*	AZD-7295
IDX-320	*MK-3281*	BMS-790052
Narlaprevir (SCH-900518)	*Nesubivr (HCV-796)*	BMS-824393
	VX-916	PPI-1301
		PPI-461
NS3 Helicase Inhibitor		**Cyclophilin Inhibitors**
BMS-650032		Alisporivir (Debio-025)
		SCY-635
		NIM-811

Italics signify compounds whose development has been halted.

Inhibitors of the NS5B polymerase are divided into two classes based upon mechanism of action: nucleoside/nucleotide analogs and non-nucleoside inhibitors. In general, this class is less potent than the NS3/4A PI class. Nucleoside/nucleotide analog inhibitors mimic the natural HCV polymerase substrate and act as chain terminators, inhibiting initiation of HCV RNA production. They are analogs of natural substrates but need to be phosphorylated for activation. They have a broader genotypic effect than NS3/4A PIs and non-nucleoside NS5B polymerase inhibitors because the NS5B active site target is highly conserved across genotypes.

Non-nucleoside inhibitors (NNIs) are allosteric inhibitors that bind with the NS5B polymerase outside of the active catalytic site and produce alterations in the protein structure that decrease its activity. The NNIs are more susceptible to development of resistance mutations because their binding sites are more distant from the NS5B active site. In addition, these sites are prone to natural polymorphisms that change conformation, and thus affect inhibitor fit and activity. NNIs have genotype activity mainly against genotype 1 (1b > 1a). There are at least four allosteric binding sites: thumb sites 1 and 2 and palm sites 1 and 2 (Legrand-Abravanel et al., 2010).

Nucleoside Analog Inhibitors

Mericitabine (RG-7128) is a potent nucleoside analog with a good safety profile and high barrier to resistance. It has a low risk of drug–drug interactions since it is excreted renally and has no significant hepatic metabolism. It has antiviral activity across genotypes 1 to 6 and no treatment-emergent viral breakthrough or resistance in initial studies (Le Pogam et al., 2010). It is being studied in two phase 2b studies, the PROPEL and JUMP-C studies. 408 genotype HCV genotype 1 or 4, treatment-naïve patients were treated with mericitabine, PEG, and RBV for 8 to 12 weeks followed by PEG/RBV for 24 to 48 weeks compared with a PEG/RBV control group. In the 1-g BID mericitabine/PEG/RBV group, RVR rates were 62% versus 18% in the control group. HCV RNA undetectable rates at 12 weeks were 80% to 87% for the mericitabine groups compared with 49% for the control group (Jensen et al., 2010). JUMP-C, an ongoing phase 2b study on HCV genotype 1 treatment-naïve patients, revealed a 76% SVR with 1g BID of mericitabine + PEG/RBV. No drug resistance was noted, although there was a 24% relapse rate (Pockros et al., 2011). As mentioned earlier, mericitabine was used with danoprevir in a PEG/RBV-sparing regimen in the INFORM trial and will be discussed later.

Other NS5B nucleoside inhibitors are under early investigation; see Table 14.1. It should be noted that several other NS5B nucleoside inhibitors have been discontinued in development, including valopicitabine (NM-283), which was stopped due to weak activity and gastrointestinal side effects, and R-1626, which was stopped due to severe lymphocytopenia associated with lethal outcomes.

Nucleotide Analog Inhibitors

PSI-7977 is a nucelotide inhibitor that is being evaluated in a phase 2b study in HCV genotypes 1, 2, and 3. In the PROTON study, 100 HCV genotype 1 treatment-naïve patients were randomized (2:2:1) to 200 mg daily of PSI-7977 + PEG/RBV versus 400 mg daily of PSI-7977 + PEG/RBV versus PEG/RBV. PSI-7977 and PEG/RBV were administered for 12 weeks with response-guided continuation of PEG/RBV for 24 or 48 weeks. 25 patients with HCV GT 2/3 were enrolled in an open label arm and treated with 12 weeks of triple therapy. The genotype 1 patients were also stratified by IL28B. In genotype 1 patients, 98% of patients in the PSI-7977 arms had RVR. At week 12, 100% in the 200-mg arm and 92% in the 400-mg arm had undetectable HCV RNA. There were no significant differences in adverse events reported between the control and PSI-7977 arms, and no viral breakthroughs were observed (Nelson et al., 2011). In the genotype 2/3 patients, 100% of those given 400 mg PSI-7977 with PEG/RBV for 12 weeks achieved SVR (Lalezari et al., 2011).

PSI-938 is another nucelotide inhibitor that was combined with PSI-7977 in the NUCLEAR study and will be discussed later.

NNI

NNI site 1 (thumb site 1)-targeted drugs under study include MK-3281, BI-207127, and BI-1941. MK-3281 is a tetracyclic indole NNI that was evaluated in 22 HCV genotype 1 and 3 patients and was found to have the highest potency against genotype 1b. Monotherapy for 7 days led to a mean decrease of 1.95 log 10 in HCV RNA, with a 3.8 log 10 drop in genotype 1b patients, compared to a 1.3 log 10 decline in genotype 1a and a 1.2 log 10 decline in genotype 3 (Brainard et al., 2009).

BI-207127 is another thumb site 1 inhibitor that was also shown to have greater activity against HCV genotype 1b than genotype 1a in a phase 1 study of 60 HCV genotype 1 treatment-naïve patients. All patients were treated for 5 days and followed for 10 to 14 days (Larrey et al., 2009).

BI-1941 was effective in decreasing HCV RNA, although gastrointestinal side effects limited treatment at higher doses. It also showed greater activity against genotype 1b compared with genotype 1a.

NNI site 2 (thumb site 2)-targeted drugs include filibuvir (PF-00868554), the most advanced site 2 NNI under development. Early studies reported up to 60% to 75% RVR in HCV genotype 1 patients given filibuvir with PEG/RBV (Jacobson et al., 2009). Interestingly, filibuvir therapy with PEG/RBV revealed more activity against HCV genotype 1a compared with 1b (Troke et al., 2009). A phase 2 study enrolling 288 HCV genotype 1 patients treated with 300 or 600 mg filibuvir with PEG/RBV is under way.

Other NNIs targeting thumb site 2 include VX-759, VX-916, and VX-222. VX-759 was studied in a phase 1, multiple ascending dose study to assess efficacy and safety in 32 patients with HCV genotype 1. The mean HCV RNA reduction was ranged from 1.97 to 2.46 log 10 for the 400-mg BID to 800-mg BID arms (Cooper et al., 2009a). A similar study was performed with VX-916 as monotherapy given to 41 subjects, revealing a maximal HCV RNA reduction of 1.5 log 10 for the highest dose arms (Lawitz et al., 2009a). VX-222 was also evaluated in a phase 1 dose-escalating study. VX-222 was well tolerated, with a mean HCV RNA reduction of more than 3 logs by day 4 (Cooper et al., 2009b; Rodriguez et al., 2010). These reports have supported phase 2 investigation for these compounds.

NNIs site 3 (palm site 1)-targeted drugs include ANA-598, ABT-333, ABT-072, and IDX-375. ANA-598 was studied in 35 subjects in a phase 1 dose-ranging study with doses from 200 mg to 800 mg twice daily compared to placebo. Median HCV RNA reductions ranged between 2.3 and 2.9 log 10 for the ANA-598 arms. There were no significant adverse events (Lawitz et al., 2009b). This led to a phase 2 study in treatment-naïve, genotype 1 patients with 12 weeks of ANA-598/PEG/RBV therapy compared to PEG/RBV, followed by 24 to 48 weeks of PEG/RBV. 42% to 56% of patients in the ANA-598 arms had an RVR compared to 13% in the PEG/RBV control group. HCV RNA was undetectable at week 12 in 73% to 75% in the ANA-598 arms compared to 63% in the controls (Lawitz et al., 2010).

In genotype 1 treatment-naïve patients, ABT-333 produced 41.7% (10/24) undetectable HCV RNA rates (HCV RNA <25 IU/mL) after 28 days of combination therapy with PEG/RBV versus 0% (0/6) in the PEG/RBV + placebo group. Side effects were described as mild and comparable to those on PEG/RBV (Rodriguez-Torres et al., 2009).

ABT-072 and IDX-375 have been shown in pharmacokinetic and replicon assay studies to be promising.

NNI site 4 (palm site 2)-targeted drugs include GS-9190. Tegobuvir (GS-9190) has a binding site close to the active site of NS5B and was developed based on the location of known resistant mutations. It was found to have significant activity in replicon systems against genotype 1. 31 HCV genotype 1, treatment-naïve patients were enrolled in a phase 1 study with doses ranging between 40 and 480 mg. HCV RNA reductions ranged between 0.7 and 1.2 log 10 at 1 day, confirming a dose-dependent efficacy (Vliegen et al., 2007). This led to a phase 2b study with PEG/RBV in 252 treatment-naïve, noncirrhotic patients with HCV genotype 1. Although RVR and extended EVR rates were higher in the tegobuvir arms compared to PEG/RBV control, SVR was similar at 56% (Lawitz et al., 2011b).

HCV-796, an NNI at site 4, was shown to have efficacy across multiple HCV genotypes as monotherapy and in combination with PEG/RBV (Pockros et al., 2007). Unfortunately, although it had strong antiviral activity, further development was halted due to significant hepatotoxicity.

NS5B inhibitors under development are shown in Table 14.1.

NS5A Inhibitors

The NS5A inhibitors are a new class of antiviral therapy that inhibits the NS5A replication complex by an unknown mechanism (Nettles et al., 2008). The first agent in this class is BMS-790052, which was found to exhibit antiviral activity against all HCV genotypes, especially genotype 1b. BMS-790052 is characterized by once-daily dosing and is well tolerated, although it is susceptible to the rapid development of resistance (Scheel et al., 2011). It was administered at three different doses with PEG/RBV and compared with placebo/PEG/RBV for 48 weeks in a phase 2a trial in 48 HCV genotype 1 treatment-naïve patients (Pol et al., 2011). SVR rates (week 12) after completion of therapy ranged between 83% and 92% in the 10-mg and 60-mg BMS-790052 arms, respectively, compared to 25% in the control group and 42% in the low-dose 3-mg BMS-790052 arm. Interestingly, subjects in the 10-mg and 60-mg groups had similar SVR rates regardless of IL28B genotype. The agent was well tolerated, with an overall side-effect profile similar to the control group. It was combined with BMS-650032, an NS3 PI, in a recent study with and without PEG/RBV and will be discussed later. Other NS5A inhibitors in evaluation include BMS-824393, AZD-7295, ABT-267, and PPI-461. Table 14.1 lists the various NS5A inhibitors under development.

NS4B Inhibitors

The function of the NS4B protein has not been well characterized, although it is thought to be associated with the formation of the vital replication complex critical to HCV replication. The RNA binding site of NS4B along the membranous web of the replication complex has become the site for drug development. No NS4B inhibitors have been studied in human studies yet, although several compounds with NS4B inhibition activity have been reported (Rai et al., 2011).

Cyclophilin Inhibitors

Alisporivir, or Debio-025, is a synthetic non-immunosuppressive form of cyclosporine that has potent and broad activity against HCV genotypes 1, 2, 3, and 4 in cell culture systems (Paeshuyse et al., 200). A phase 2 dose-ranging trial (200 mg to 1,000 mg BID) involved 90 HCV treatment-naïve subjects divided into five groups for 29 days (Flisiak et al., 2009). Debio-025 provided a dose-dependent effect with HCV RNA reduction between 2.2 and 4.75 log 10. A follow-up study of PEG/RBV treatment in these patients revealed an SVR of 67% without significant toxicity related to Debio-025 (Flisiak et al., 2010). However, initial reports of the phase 2a trial conducted on 50 HCV genotype 1 nonresponders to PEG/RBV showed no significant HCV RNA reduction, leading to questions regarding its true efficacy and the need for a loading dose or higher dose (Nelson et al., 2009). Also, mild conjugated hyperbilirubinemia was noted in some patients. A phase 2b, double-blind, placebo-controlled trial is ongoing. Of import, in vitro studies of Debio-025 reported a lack of significant cross-resistance with NS3/4A PIs or the NS5B polymerase inhibitors, suggesting its potential importance in future combination therapy regimens (Coelmont et al., 2009).

SCY-635 is another cyclophilin inhibitor under investigation (Hopkins et al., 2010a). 20 patients with HCV genotype 1 were treated with 300 to 900 mg SCY-635 for 15 days in a phase 1 study. In the 900-mg dosing cohort, a mean decline of 2.3 log 10 HCV RNA was noted. There was no significant toxicity (Hopkins et al., 2009). Resistance testing showed a high barrier to resistance without treatment-associated mutations resulting in virologic breakthrough (Hopkins et al., 2010b). A phase 2a trial in HCV genotype 1 treatment-naïve patients is ongoing.

The development of another cyclophilin inhibitor, NIM-811, was stopped due to concerns regarding hyperbilirubinemia and thrombocytopenia (Lawitz et al., 2009c).

Miscellaneous

HCV entry inhibitors that target host cell surface molecules such as IDX-320, IDX-375, and REP-9C have yet to progress to phase 2 studies. Alpha-glucosidase inhibitors that lead to misfolding of the HCV envelope protein, blocking viral assembly and release, have also been evaluated. Celgosivir (MX-3235) has been studied in the most detail and, unfortunately, has been ineffective (Yoshida et al., 2006).

Combination Therapy

Although the addition of boceprevir or telaprevir to PEG/RBV has dramatically increased SVR in patients with HCV genotype 1, efficacy is still limited. Many patients have contraindications to PEG and/or RBV and will not be candidates to receive the current regimen. There are many drug–drug interactions with the current PIs that limit usage of the regimen. The current PIs used without complementary DAAs also may lead to the development of resistance-associated mutations. In fact, even in the select patient populations in clinical trials, 21% to 34% of patients did not achieve SVR. African American and cirrhotic populations do less well. Therefore, there is an impetus to combine DAAs to offer interferon-free regimens with high SVR and excellent tolerability. Furthermore, it is possible that the addition of highly effective DAA combinations with PEG and RBV may increase the efficacy of PEG and RBV and yield increased SVR with a quadruple regimen. HCV has mechanisms that inhibit the immune response; for instance, the NS3 protease inactivates host proteins that modulate innate interferon-modulated immunity. It is possible that lower viral levels from potent viral replication inhibition without the development of resistance and inhibition of NS3 in particular may increase the efficacy of the regimen.

DAA combinations are chosen based upon providing complementary mechanisms of action that will avoid cross-resistance, minimize drug–drug interactions, and reduce overlapping toxicities. Table 14.2 lists the various combination DAA regimens under investigation.

Table 14.2 DAA Combination Studies

DAA #1: NS3/4A PI	DAA #2
Danoprevir (RG-7227/ ITMN-191)	Mericitabine (RG-7128) (NS5B polymerase inhibitor)
BMS-650032	BMS-790052 (NS5A inhibitor)
BI-201335	BI-207127 (Non-nucleoside NS5B polymerase inhibitor)
GS-9256	Tegobuvir (GS-9190) (Non-nucleoside NS5B polymerase inhibitor)
Telaprevir	VX-222 (Non-nucleoside NS5B polymerase inhibitor)
IDX-320	IDX-184 (NS5a inhibitor)
ABT-450	ABT-072 (Non-nucleoside NS5B polymerase inhibitor)

The INFORM 1 study was a randomized, placebo-controlled, double-blinded trial involving 88 HCV genotype 1 patients including both treatment-naïve and -experienced subjects. Patients were administered different doses of mericitabine (RG-7128), an NS5B polymerase inhibitor, and danoprevir (RG-7227/ ITMN-191), an NS3/4A PI, versus placebo for 14 days without PEG or RBV. The median HCV RNA reduction was 3.7 to 5.2 log 10. 88% of subjects receiving the highest doses of both mericitabine and danoprevir had undetectable HCV RNA at day 14. The combination was well tolerated and was a proof of concept that an oral combination regimen could yield potent viral suppression without significant toxicity or development of high rates of resistance over the short term (Gane et al., 2010).

BMS-790052 (NS5A inhibitor) and BMS-650032 (NS3 PI) with or without PEG/RBV for 24 weeks in HCV genotype 1, noncirrhotic, null responders to PEG/RBV was recently reported (Lok et al., 2011). Eleven patients were administered combination therapy without PEG/RBV and 10 were given quadruple therapy. Four of 11 patients (2/2 genotype 1b, 2/9 genotype 1a) in the PEG/RBV-free arm achieved SVR, supporting the concept that PEG/RBV-free combination DAA regimens can yield SVR. Furthermore, all 10 patients given quadruple therapy had end-of-treatment response, and undetectable HCV RNA 12 weeks after treatment completion. Nine of 10 patients had SVR. This supported the concept that DAAs may increase PEG/RBV sensitivity since all of the patients were previously null responders to PEG/RBV. Most adverse events were mild to moderate in severity, and there were no serious adverse events or treatment discontinuations. Six patients in the dual combination therapy group had HCV RNA breakthrough and were found to have resistance to BMS-790052 and BMS-650032. However, the initiation of PEG/RBV in these patients led to HCV RNA suppression, leaving four patients with undetectable HCV RNA levels.

Combination BI-201335 (NS3/4A PI) with BI-207127 (NS5B polymerase inhibitor) therapy was also studied in conjunction with RBV in the SOUND-C1 and SOUND-C2 studies in PEG-free regimens. 32 treatment-naïve, genotype 1 patients were treated over 4 weeks with 120 mg daily of BI-201335, 400 or 600 mg TID of BI207127, and 1,000/1,200 mg daily in two doses of RBV. By day 29, 73% of the 400-mg TID BI-207127 group and 100% of the 600-mg TID group had undetectable HCV RNA. However, two patients with genotype 1a in the lower-dose 400-mg TID group had viral rebound during treatment (Zeuzem et al., 2010).

Two NS5B polymerase inhibitors, PSI-7977 and PSI-938, were given over 14 days to 32 HCV genotype 1 treatment-naïve patients in the NUCLEAR study that evaluated the safety, efficacy, pharmacokinetics, and interaction between the two compounds. A mean 5 log 10 HCV RNA reduction was observed in the combination arms without appearance of significant resistance (Lawitz et al., 2011c).

Tegobuvir (GS-9190), an NS5B polymerase inhibitor, and GS-9256, an NS3/4A PI, with or without PEG and/or RBV was studied. GS-9256 is under phase 2 development currently, with only phase 1 clinical data available for monotherapy (Goldwater et al, 2010). 46 subjects were enrolled. 100% achieved RVR with quadruple therapy compared to 38% with GS-9190/GS-9256/RBV and 7% with GS-9190/GS-9256 alone. At week 24, the HCV RNA undetectable rates were 100%, 100%, and 67%, respectively. GS-9190 and GS-9256 were well tolerated and associated with decreased emergence of resistance-associated mutations. This study indicated that RBV is beneficial even in the absence of PEG (Foster et al., 2011).

A combination trial with TMC-435, an NS3/4A PI, with PSI-7977, an NS5B polymerase inhibitor, with or without RBV in prior null responders to PEG/RBV is also under way.

Conclusion

Although the approval of the two new NS3/4A PI, boceprevir and telaprevir, is an important milestone in the treatment of HCV, the excitement must be tempered by the recognition of limitations and risks. In the future, highly effective, well-tolerated regimens are sought. Shorter courses of therapy that work for all genotypes would be ideal. Favorable dosing regimens with minimal drug–drug interactions would be optimal. A therapeutic regimen that is effective in difficult-to-treat populations is important (Table 14.3). Interferon-free regimens may provide the best opportunity to achieve these goals. Fortunately, there are

Table 14.3 Groups Not Accommodated by PIs	
Patients with Contraindications to PEG/RBV	**Patients NOT Studied with PIs**
Women who are or may become pregnant	Non-genotype 1: genotypes 2 to 6
Men whose female partners are pregnant	Pediatric patients
Major neuropsychiatric disease	Human immunodeficiency virus co-infection
Major coronary or cerebrovascular disease	Hepatitis B co-infection
Active substance or alcohol abuse	Solid organ transplant recipients
Allergy to PEG or RBV	Moderate/severe hepatic impairment (Child-Pugh B/C or score >=7)
	Decompensated liver disease

numerous promising DAA agents under investigation. In the near future, it is likely that some of these compounds will emerge as therapeutic options for HCV that further improve treatment of this deadly disease.

References

Armstrong, G. L., A. Wasley, E. P. Simard, et al. (2006). The prevalence of hepatitis C virus infection in the United States, 1999 through 2002. *Annals of Internal Medicine, 144*(10), 705–714.

Brainard, D. A., M. S. Anderson, A. Petry, et al. (2009). Safety and antiviral activity of NS5B polymerase inhibitor MK–3281, in treatment-naïve genotype 1A, 1B and 3 HCV–infected patients. *Hepatology, 50*, 1026A–1027A.

Bronowicki, J. P., S. Pol, P. J. Thuluvath, et al. (2011). BMS–650032, an NS3 inhibitor, in combination with peginterferon alpha-2a and ribavirin in treatment-naïve subjects with genotype 1 chronic hepatitis C infection. *Journal of Hepatology, 54*(S1), S472.

Cheng, K. C., S. Gupta, H. Wang, et al. (2011). Current drug discovery strategies for treatment of hepatitis C virus infection. *Journal of Pharmacy & Pharmacology, 63*(7), 883–892.

Coelmont, L., S. Kaptein, J. Paeshuyse, et al. (2009). Debio 025, a cyclophilin binding molecule, is highly efficient in clearing hepatitis C virus (HCV) replicon-containing cells when used alone or in combination with specifically targeted antiviral therapy for HCV (STAT–C) inhibitors. *Antimicrobial Agents Chemotherapy, 53*, 967–976.

Cooper, C., E. J. Lawitz, P. Ghali, et al. (2009a). Evaluation of VCH–759 monotherapy in hepatitis C infection. *Journal of Hepatology, 51*(1), 39–46.

Cooper, C., R. Larouche, B. Bourgault, et al. (2009b). Safety, tolerability and pharmacokinetics of the HCV polymerase inhibitor VCH–222 following single dose administration in healthy volunteers and antiviral activity in HCV-infected individuals. *Journal of Hepatology, 50*, S342.

Detishin, V., W. Haazen, R. Hooijmaijers, et al. (2011). Final results of the pharmacokinetics, efficacy, and safety/tolerability of 400 and 600 mg once-daily dosing of ACH–1625 (HCV NS3 protease inhibitor) in HCV genotype 1. *Journal of Hepatology, 54*(S1), S186–187.

Flisiak, R., S. V. Feinman, M. Jablkowski, et al. (2009). The cyclophilin inhibitor Debio 025 combined with PEG IFN alpha2a significantly reduces viral load in treatment–naïve hepatitis C patients. *Hepatology, 49*(5), 1460–1468.

Flisiak, R., M. Woynarowski, M. Jablkowski, et al. (2010). Efficacy of standard of care therapy following experimental DEBIO 025 treatment in patients with chronic hepatitis C. *Journal of Hepatology, 52*, S291.

Forestier, N., D. Larrey, D. Guyader, et al. (2011). Treatment of chronic hepatitis C patients with the NS3/4A protease inhibitor danoprevir (ITMN–191/RG7227) leads to robust reductions in viral RNA, A phase 1b multiple ascending dose study. *Journal of Hepatology, 54*(6), 1130–1136.

Foster, G. R., P. Buggisch, P. Marcellin, et al. (2011). Four-week treatment with GS–9256 and tegobuvir (GS–9190), ± RBV ± PEG, results in enhanced viral suppression on follow-up PEG/RBV therapy, in genotype 1A/1B HCV patients. *Journal of Hepatology, 54*(S1), S172.

Fried, M. W., M. L. Shiffman, K. R. Reddy, et al. (2002). Peginterferon alfa-2a plus ribavirin for chronic hepatitis C virus infection. *New England Journal of Medicine, 347*(13), 975–982.

Fried, M. W., M. Buti, G. J. Dore, et al. (2010). Efficacy and safety of TMC435 in combination with peginteferon alfa-2A and ribavirin in treatment-naïve genotype 1 HCV patients, 24 week interim results from the PILLAR study. *Hepatology, 52,* 107A.

Gane, E. J., S. K. Roberts, C. A. Stedman, et al. (2010).Oral combination therapy with a nucleoside polymerase inhibitor (RG7128) and danoprevir for chronic hepatitis C genotype 1 infection (INFORM–1), a randomised, double-blind, placebo-controlled, dose-escalation trial. *Lancet, 376*(9751), 1467–1475.

Goldwater, R., M. P. DeMicco, J. Zong J, et al. (2010). Safety, pharmacokinetics, and antiviral activity of single oral doses of the HCV NS3 protease inhibitor GS 9256. *Hepatology, 52,* 717A.

Hezode, C., N. Forestier, G. Dusheiko, et al. (2009). Telaprevir and peginterferon with or without ribavirin for chronic HCV infection. *New England Journal of Medicine, 360,* 1839–1850.

Hopkins, S., D. Heuman, E. Gavis, et al. (2009). Safety, plasma pharmacokinetics and anti–viral activity of SCY–635 in adult patients with chronic hepatitis C virus infection. *Journal of Hepatology, 50,* S36.

Hopkins, S., B. Scorneaux, Z. Huang, et al. (2010a). SCY–635, a novel nonimmunosuppressive analog of cyclosporine that exhibits potent inhibition of hepatitis C virus RNA replication in vitro. *Antimicrobial Agents Chemotherapy, 54,* 660–672.

Hopkins, S., S. Mosier, R. Harris, et al. (2010b). Resistance selection following 15 days of monotherapy with SCY–635 a non-immunosuppressive cyclophilin inhibitor with potent anti–HCV activity. *Journal of Hepatology, 52,* S15.

Jacobson, I., P. Pockros, J. Lalezari, et al. (2009). Antiviral activity of filibuvir in combination with pegylated inteferon alfa–2a and ribavirin for 28 days in treatment naive patients chronically infected with HCV genotype 1. *Journal of Hepatology, 50,* S382–383.

Jensen, D. M., H. Wedemeyer, R. W. Herring, et al. (2010). High rates of early viral response, promising safety profile and lack resistance-related breakthrough in HCV GT1/4 patients treated with RG7128 plus pegIFN alfa–2a (40KD)/RBV, planned week 12 interim analysis from the PROPEL study. *Hepatology, 52,* 360–361A.

Lalezari, J., E. Lawitz, M. Rodriguez–Torres, et al. (2011). Once daily PSI-7977 plus PEGIFN/RBV in a phase 2B trial, rapid virological suppression in treatment-naïve patients with HCV GT2/GT3. *Journal of Hepatology, 54*(S1), S28.

Larrey, D. G., Y. Benhamou, A. W. Lohse, et al. (2009). BI 207127 is a potent HCV RNA polymerase inhibitor during 5 days monotherapy in patients with chronic hepatitis C. *Hepatology, 50,* 1044A.

Lawitz, E., C. Cooper, M. Rodriguez–Torres, et al. (2009a). Safety, tolerability and antiviral activity of VCH–916, a novel non–nucleoside HCV polymerase inhibitor in patients with chronic HCV genotype 1 infection. *Journal of Hepatology, 50,* S37.

Lawitz, E., M. Rodriguez–Torres, M. DeMicco, et al. (2009b). Antiviral activity of ANA598, a potent non–nucleoside polymerase inhibitor, in chronic hepatitis C patients. *Journal of Hepatology, 50,* S384.

Lawitz, E., R. Rouzier, T. Nguyen, et al. (2009c). Safety and antiviral efficacy of 14 days of the cyclophilin inhibitor NIM811 in combination with pegylated inteferon alpha 2a in relapsed genotype I HCV infected patients. *Journal of Hepatology, 50*, S379.

Lawitz, E., M. Rodriguez–Torres, V. K. Rustgi, et al. (2010). Safety and antiviral activity of ANA598 in combination with pegylated interferon alfa–2A plus ribavirin in treatment-naive genotype 1 chronic HCV patients. *Hepatology, 52*, 334A–335A.

Lawitz, E., I. Gaultier, F. Poordad, et al. (2011a). ABT–450/Ritonavir (ABT–450/R) combined with pegylated interferon alpha-2a and ribavirin (SOC) after 30-day monotherapy in genotype 1 HCV-infected treatment-naïve subjects, 120-week interim efficacy and safety results. *Journal of Hepatology, 54*(S1), S482.

Lawitz, E., I. Jacobson, E. Godofsky, et al. (2011b). A phase 2B trial comparing 24 to 48 weeks treatment with tegobuvir (GS–9190)/PEG/RBV to 48 weeks treatment with PEG/RBV for chronic genotype 1 HCV infection. *Journal of Hepatology, 54*(S1), S181.

Lawitz, E., M. Rodriguez–Torres, J. Denning, et al. (2011c). Once daily dual-nucleotide combination of PSI–938 and PSI–7977 provides 94% HCV RNA < LOD at day 14, first purine/pyrimidine clinical combination data (the NUCLEAR study). *Journal of Hepatology, 54*(S1), S543.

Legrand-Abravanel, F., F. Nicot, & J. Izopet (2010). New NS5B polymerase inhibitors for hepatitis C. *Expert Opinion Investigational Drugs, 19*(8), 963–975.

Le Pogam, S., A. Seshaadri, A. Ewing, et al. (2010). RG7128 alone or in combination with pegylated interferon–α2a and ribavirin prevents hepatitis C virus (HCV) Replication and selection of resistant variants in HCV-infected patients. *Journal of Infectious Disease, 202*, 1510–1519.

Liu, Z., F. Yang, J. M. Robotham, et al. (2009). Critical role of cyclophilin A and its prolyl–peptidyl isomerase activity in the structure and function of the hepatitis C virus replication complex. *Journal of Virology, 83*, 6554–6565.

Lok, A. S., D. F. Gardiner, E. Lawitz, et al. (2011). Quadruple therapy with BMS–790052, BMS–650032 and PEG-IFN/RBV for 24 weeks; results in 100% SVR12 in HCV genotype 1 null responders. *Journal of Hepatology, 54*(S1), S536.

Manns, M. P., J. G. McHutchison, S. C. Gordon, et al. (2001). Peginterferon alfa-2b plus ribavirin compared with interferon alfa-2b plus ribavirin for initial treatment of chronic hepatitis C, a randomised trial. *Lancet, 358*(9286), 958–965.

Manns, M. P., E. J. Gane, M. Rodriguez-Torres, et al. (2010). Sustained viral response (SVR) rates in genotype 1 treatment-naïve patients with chronic hepatitis C (CHC) infection treated with vaniprevir (MK–7009), a NS3/4A protease inhibitor, in combination with pegylated interferon alfa-2A and ribavirin for 28 days. *Hepatology, 52*, 361A.

Manns, M. P., M. Bourlière, Y. Benhamou, et al. (2011). Potency, safety, and pharmacokinetics of the NS3/4A protease inhibitor BI201335 in patients with chronic HCV genotype 1 infection. *Journal of Hepatology, 54*(6), 1114–1122.

Nelson, D. R., R. H. Ghalib, M. Sulkowski, et al. (2009). Efficacy and safety of the cyclophilin inhibitor Debio 025 in combination with pegylated interferon alpha-2a and ribavirin in previously null-responder genotype 1 HCV patients. *Journal of Hepatology, 50*, S40.

Nelson, D. R., J. Lalezari, E. Lawitz, et al. (2011). Once daily PSI-7977 plus PEG-IFN/RBV in HCV GT1, 98% rapid virological response, complete early virological response, the PROTON study. *Journal of Hepatology, 54*(S1), S544.

Nettles, R., C. Chien, E. Chung, et al. (2008). BMS-790052 is a first-in-class potent hepatitis C virus (HCV) NS5A inhibitor for patients with chronic HCV infection, results from a proof-of-concept study. *Hepatology, 48*, 1025A.

Paeshuyse, J., A. Kaul, E. De Clercq, et al. (2006). The non-immunosuppressive cyclosporin DEBIO-025 is a potent inhibitor of hepatitis C virus replication in vitro. *Hepatology, 43*, 761–770.

Pockros, P., M. Rodriguez-Torres, S. Villano, et al. (2007). A phase 2, randomized study of HCV–796 in combination with pegylated interferon (PEG) plus ribavirin (RBV) versus PEG plus RBV in hepatitis C virus genotype 1 infection. *Journal of Hepatology, 56*, S7–8.

Pockros, P., D. Jensen, N. Tsai, et al. (2011). First SVR data with the nucleoside analogue polymerase inhibitor mericitabine (RG7128) combined with peginterferon/ribavirin in treatment-naïve HCV G1/4 patients, interim analysis from the JUMP-C trial. *Journal of Hepatology, 54*(S1), S538.

Pol, S., R. H. Ghalib, V. K. Rustgi, et al. (2011). First report of SVR12 for a NS5A replication complex inhibitor BMS–790052 in combination with PEG-IFNa-2a and RBV, phase 2a trial in treatment-naive HCV genotype 1 subjects. *Journal of Hepatology, 54*(S1), S544–545.

Rai, R., & J. Deval (2011). New opportunities in anti-hepatitis C virus drug discovery, targeting NS4B. *Antiviral Research, 90*(2), 93–101.

Reesink, H. W., G. C. Fanning, K. A. Farha, et al. (2010). Rapid HCV-RNA decline with once daily TMC435, a phase I study in healthy volunteers and hepatitis C patients. *Gastroenterology, 138*(3), 913–921.

Rodriguez-Torres, M., E. Lawitz, D. Cohen, et al. (2009). Treatment-naive, HCV genotype 1-infected subjects show significantly greater HCV RNA decreases when treated with 28 days of ABT-333 plus peginterferon and ribavirin compared to peginterferon and ribavirin alone. *Hepatology, 50*, 5A.

Rodriguez, M., E. Lawitz, B. Conway, et al. (2010). Safety and antiviral activity of the HCV non–nucleoside polymerase inhibitor VX-222 in treatment-naïve genotype 1 HCV-infected patients. *Journal of Hepatology, 52*, S14.

Rouzier, R., D. Larrey, E. J. Gane, et al. (2011). Activity of danoprevir plus low-dose ritonavir (DNV/R) in combination with peginterferon alfa-2a (40KD) plus ribavirin (PEGIFNa-2a/RBV) in previous null responders. *Journal of Hepatology, 54*(S1), S28.

Scheel, T. K., J. M. Gottwein, L. S. Mikkelsen, et al. (2011). Recombinant HCV variants with NS5A from genotypes 1–7 have different sensitivities to an NS5A inhibitor but not interferon-α. *Gastroenterology, 140*(3), 1032–1042.

Sklan, E. H., P. Charuworn, P. S. Pang, et al. (2009). Mechanisms of HCV survival in the host. *Nature Reviews Gastroenterology Hepatology, 6*(4), 217–227.

Sulkowski, M. S., E. Ceasu, T. Asselah, et al. (2011a). SILEN-C1, Sustained virological response (SVR) and safety of BI201335 combined with peginterferon alfa-2a and ribavirin (P/R) in treatment-naïve patients with chronic genotype 1 HCV infection. *Journal of Hepatology, 54*(S1), S27.

Sulkowski, M. S., M. Bourliere, J. P. Bronowicki, et al. (2011b). SILEN-C2, Sustained virological response (SVR) and safety of BI201335 combined with peginterferon alfa-2a and ribavirin (P/R) in chronic HCV genotype 1 patients with nonresponse to P/R. *Journal of Hepatology, 54*(S1), S30.

Terrault, N., C. Cooper, L. A. Balart, et al. (2010). Phase II randomised, partially-blind, parallel-group study of oral danoprevir (RG7227) with PEGIFN alfa-2A (Pegasys) plus ribavirin in treatment-naive genotype 1 patients with CHC, results of planned week 12 interim analysis of the ATLAS study. *Hepatology, 52*, 335A–336A.

Troke, P., M. Lewis, P. Simpson, et al. (2009). Genotypic characterization of HCV NS5B following 8-day monotherapy with the polymerase inhibitor PF-00868554 in HCV-infected subjects. *Journal of Hepatology, 50*, S351.

Watashi, K., N. Ishii, M. Hijikata, et al. (2005). Cyclophilin B is a functional regulator of hepatitis C virus RNA polymerase. *Molecular Cell, 19*, 111–122.

Vliegen, I., J. Paeshuyse, E. Marbery, et al. (2007). GS–9190, a novel substituted imidazopyridine analogue, is a potent inhibitor of hepatitis C virus replication in vitro and remains active against known drug resistant mutants. *Hepatology, 46*, 855A.

Yoshida, E., D. Kunimoto, S. S. Lee, et al. (2006). Results of a phase 2 dose ranging study of orally administered celgosivir as monotherapy in chronic hepatitis C genotype 1 patients. *Gastroenterology, 130*, A784.

Zeuzem, S., T. Asselah, P. W. Angus, et al. (2010). Strong antiviral activity and safety of IFN–sparing treatment with the protease inhibitor BI 201335, the HCV polymerase inhibitor BI 207127 and ribavirin in patients with chronic hepatitis C. *Hepatology, 52*, 876A.

Zeuzem, S., G. R. Foster, M. W. Fried, et al. (2011). The ASPIRE trial, TMC435 in treatment-experienced patients with genotype 1 HCV infection who have failed previous PEGIFN/RBV treatment. *Journal of Hepatology, 54*(S1), S546.

Chapter 15

Lexicon of Trials for Treatment of Chronic Hepatitis C

Archita P. Desai and Nancy Reau

Hoofnagle et al, NEJM, (1986). Treatment of Chronic Non-A, Non-B Hepatitis with Recombinant Human Alpha Interferon

Study Design

Ten patients who were thought to have non-A, non-B hepatitis with changes on liver biopsy consistent with chronic hepatitis (three with cirrhosis) and persistently elevated serum aminotransferase levels were treated with alpha interferon (alfa-2b) subcutaneously 4 to 5 million IU every other day or three times a week with "gradual" dose reductions based on changes in serum aminotransferase levels and side effects.

Key Findings

First study to look at use of alpha interferon for treatment of non-A, non-B hepatitis, with eight out of ten patients experiencing a dramatic decrease in serum aminotransferase levels while on therapy. Findings also supported that prolonged therapy would be needed for sustained benefit. Side effects were fatigue, achiness, headaches, irritability, and fever.

Davis et al, NEJM, (1989). Treatment of Chronic Hepatitis C with Recombinant Interferon Alfa: a multicenter randomized, controlled trial

Study Design

166 patients at 12 centers with presumed chronic hepatitis C (received blood transfusion or had exposure to blood with persistently elevated aminotransferase levels and liver biopsy showing chronic hepatitis) were randomly assigned to three groups: no treatment versus recombinant interferon alfa-2b 1 million IU versus 3 million IU three times per week for 24 weeks. Patients were followed for up to 46 weeks after completion of therapy. 86% of patients had positive antibody to the hepatitis C virus and 55% of patients had cirrhosis.

Key Findings

Complete response (defined by normal serum aminotransferase levels) was achieved in 38% of patients receiving higher-dose interferon alfa-2b versus 16% in the low-dose group versus 4% in the non-treatment group. Paired liver biopsies were available for 84% of patients, with histologic improvement in 52% of the patients in the high-dose group versus 29% in the low-dose group. After treatment was discontinued, sustained response was noted in 52% of patients during the follow-up period, with relapse noted in about 50% of both treatment groups. Side effects were noted in all three groups at similar rates and included nausea, irritability, and depression, although flu-like symptoms occurred more frequently in patients treated with interferon.

Lai et al, Gastroenterology, (1996). Long-term efficacy of ribavirin plus interferon alfa in the treatment of chronic hepatitis C

Study Design

60 patients with chronic hepatitis C in Taiwan without cirrhosis and no prior therapy were assigned to three groups: interferon alfa-2a 3 million IU three times weekly plus ribavirin 1,200 mg daily versus interferon alone versus no therapy for 24 weeks. All patients were followed for 2 years.

Key Findings

At the end of a 24-week treatment period, 76% of patients in the combination therapy group had normalized ALT compared to 37% in the group treated with interferon alone versus 10% in the untreated group. Sustained response, as measured by clearance of HCV viremia at the end of the 2-year follow-up period, was also higher in the combination therapy group, 43% versus 6%. Rapid virologic and biochemical response within 2 weeks of starting therapy was noted in those patients who went on to achieve sustained virologic response. Patients with genotype 1b HCV infection had a trend towards a lower response rate in the combination therapy group (36% vs. 57%). Adverse effects were more frequent in the treatment groups, with an increased incidence of "mild" anemia, leukopenia, and indirect hyperbilirubinemia in patients receiving combination therapy, with 10% of patients requiring dose reduction of ribavirin due to anemia. In conclusion, this is the first study of combination therapy with ribavirin and interferon alfa and shows that combination therapy can induce sustained normalization of ALT levels and clearance of HCV RNA in 43% of noncirrhotic patients.

McHutchison et al, NEJM, (1998). Interferon alfa-2b alone or in combination with ribavirin as initial treatment for chronic hepatitis C

Study Design

Randomized, double-blind, placebo-controlled U.S. trial to evaluate the safety and efficacy of interferon alfa-2b alone and in combination with ribavirin.

Patients were assigned to four groups: interferon alfa-2b plus placebo for 24 weeks or 48 weeks versus the combination of interferon alfa-2b and ribavirin for 24 weeks or 48 weeks. The dosage of interferon for all groups was 3 million units three times subcutaneously per week; for ribavirin the dosage was 1,000 to 1,200 mg twice a day.

Key Findings

SVR rates were higher among the patients who received interferon and ribavirin (31% to 38%) compared to interferon alone (13%). SVR rates after combination therapy were higher after 48 weeks (38%) versus after 24 weeks (31%). Relapse was less common after 48 weeks of combination therapy versus interferon alone (42% vs. 80% at week 24). Interestingly, in this study RVR was not associated with SVR, with 59% of patients achieving SVR having HCV RNA until week 12 or week 24 of therapy. Most patients who achieved SVR also experienced normalization of serum ALT levels (88%). In addition, the histologic response was strongest in the combination therapy group treated for 48 weeks. Of the patients achieving SVR, 86% had a decrease in hepatic inflammation versus only 39% of patients who were still viremic at the end of therapy. Patients with genotype 1 infection benefited most from combination therapy for 48 weeks, with SVR rates of 28% compared to 16% after 24 weeks of therapy. Patients with genotype 2 or 3 infection gained little benefit from a longer duration of therapy, with similar SVR rates for 24 or 48 weeks of therapy. Variables associated with SVR included combination therapy, therapy for 48 weeks, HCV genotype other than 1, baseline viral load below 2 million copies/mL, female sex, and absence of cirrhosis at baseline. Adverse events included anemia requiring dose reductions in 8% of patients, but longer duration of therapy did not significantly increase dose reduction or discontinuation rates. Dyspnea, pharyngitis, pruritus, rash, nausea, insomnia, and anorexia were more common in combination therapy, and the most common reason for discontinuation in all four groups was emotional disturbance. In conclusion, combination therapy with interferon alfa-2b and ribavirin for 24 or 48 weeks is superior to interferon alone, is relatively safe, with minor increases in the need of dose reduction, and is therefore indicated as initial therapy for patients with chronic hepatitis C.

Zeuzem et al, NEJM, (2000). **Peginterferon alfa-2a in patients with chronic hepatitis C**

Study Design

In this phase 3, randomized, open-label international trial, interferon-naïve patients with chronic hepatitis C were randomly assigned to receive either peginterferon alfa-2a 180 µg/week for 48 weeks or interferon alfa-2a 6 million units three times a week for 12 weeks and then 3 million units three times a week for 36 weeks. Patients were followed for a total of 72 weeks (48 weeks on treatment and 24 weeks after completion of therapy).

Key Findings

Both end-of-treatment response and SVR rates were higher in the group treated with pegylated interferon (ETR 69% vs. 28% and SVR 39% vs. 19%), but relapse rates between 48 weeks and 72 weeks were higher in the peginterferon group. A multiple logistic regression model looking at demographic and baseline characteristics found that younger age (≤40 years), smaller body-surface area (≤2 m²), lower level of HCV RNA (≤2 million copies/mL), higher ALT level, absence of cirrhosis or bridging fibrosis, and non-genotype 1 HCV infection were associated with higher odds of a SVR. The frequency and safety of adverse outcomes were similar in the two groups. Rates of discontinuation of therapy and dose modification were similar between the two groups (7% vs. 10% and 19% vs. 18% respectively). In conclusion, peginterferon alfa-2a is safe and more effective in the treatment of chronic hepatitis C than interferon alfa-2a alone.

Manns et al, Lancet, (2001). **Peginterferon alpha-2b plus Ribavirin compared with Interferon alpha-2b plus ribavirin for initial treatment of chronic hepatitis C: a randomised trial**

Study Design

In this randomized, open-label international trial, treatment-naïve patients were randomized to three groups: (1) peginterferon alfa-2b 1.5 μg/kg subcutaneously weekly plus oral ribavirin at a flat dose of 800 mg/day for 48 weeks (high-dose peginterferon group); (2) peginterferon alfa-2b subcutaneously at a dose of 1.5 μg/kg each week for the first 4 weeks followed by 0.5 μg/kg per week for the next 44 weeks plus weight-based dose of 1,000 to 1,200 mg/day of ribavirin orally for 48 weeks (low-dose peginterferon group); and (3) interferon alfa-2b (Intron A, Schering Corp.), 3 million units subcutaneously three times per week, plus weight-based dose of 1,000 to 1,200 mg/day of ribavirin orally, both for 48 weeks (interferon group).

Key Findings

The SVR rate was higher for the higher-dose peginterferon group (54%) versus the lower-dose peginterferon group (47%) versus the interferon group (47%), with the benefits of higher-dose peginterferon most notable for genotype 1 patients. HCV genotype other than genotype 1, lower baseline viral load, lower baseline weight, younger age, and absence of bridging fibrosis were associated with SVR. Logistic regression analysis showed a strong linear relationship between ribavirin exposure (in mg/kg) and SVR in the high-dose peginterferon/flat-dose ribavirin group, suggesting that superior SVR rates (up to 61%) would be attainable if a higher dose of ribavirin than the 800-mg/day dosage had been used. Side-effect profiles between the three groups were similar, but rates of influenza-like symptoms and injection site reactions were higher in the high-dose peginterferon group. Anemia and neutropenia occurred in 9% and 18% of patients in the high-dose peginterferon group versus 13% and 8% in the interferon group, respectively, but treatment discontinuation for anemia or neutropenia was rare. In conclusion, in this large randomized study, treatment with peginterferon alfa-2b µg/kg weekly in combination with ribavirin for 48 weeks significantly increased SVR rates and lowered relapse rates and should be considered the standard of care for patients with chronic hepatitis C.

Fried et al, NEJM, (2002). **Peginterferon alfa-2a plus Ribavirin for Chronic Hepatitis C Virus Infection**

Study Design

In this randomized, open-label trial by the Pegasys International Study Group, treatment-naïve patients were randomized to three groups: (1) peginterferon alfa-2a 180 µg/wk plus ribavirin 1,000 to 1,200 mg daily; (2) peginterferon alfa-2a 180 µg/wk; (3) interferon alfa-2b 3 million units 3 times/wk plus ribavirin 1,000 to 1, 200 mg daily. Treatment duration was 48 weeks for all groups.

Key Findings

Patients treated with peginterferon alfa-2a plus weight-based ribavirin had higher SVR rates than those treated with interferon alfa-2b plus ribavirin (56% vs. 44%) or peginterferon alfa-2a alone (56% vs. 29%). For genotype 1, SVR was achieved in 46% versus 36% versus 21%, respectively. HCV genotype other than 1, age 40 years or less, and body weight less than 75 kg significantly increased the odds of SVR in patients who received peginterferon alfa-2a plus ribavirin. Most patients (97%) who did not achieve a virologic response by week 12 (early virologic response) were unlikely to achieve an SVR. The proportion of patients withdrawn from treatment because of adverse events were similar in the three groups. Cytopenias were more severe in the groups receiving peginterferon plus ribavirin but were not associated with serious sequelae and were managed with dose reduction. Patients treated with peginterferon alfa-2a had a lower incidence of influenza-like symptoms and depression. In conclusion, peginterferon alfa-2a significantly improves SVR rates for all patients with chronic hepatitis C when used in combination with ribavirin. In addition, prediction of SVR based on absence of response at week 12 may allow patients who are unlikely to respond to further therapy to stop treatment and avoid adverse events.

Hadziyannis et al, Ann Intern Med, (2004). **Peginterferon alfa-2a and Ribavirin Combination Therapy in Chronic Hepatitis C**

Study Design

In this phase 3, randomized, double-blind trial by the Pegasys International Study Group, treatment-naïve patients were randomized to four groups: (1) peginterferon alfa-2a 180 ug/wk plus ribavirin 800 mg/d for 24 weeks (24-LD);

(2) peginterferon alfa-2a plus ribavirin 1,000 to 1,200 mg/d for 24 weeks (24-SD); (3) peginterferon alfa-2a plus ribavirin 800 mg/d for 48 weeks (48-LD); (4) peginterferon alfa-2a plus ribavirin 1,000 to 1,200 mg/d for 48 weeks (48-SD).

Key Findings

Longer treatment with weight-based ribavirin improved SVR rates. When results were stratified for genotype 1 versus 2 or 3 and low versus high viral load, patients with genotype 1 had the highest response in the group treated for 48 weeks (OR 2.19) and with weight-based ribavirin (OR 1.55), with an SVR of 52% in patients receiving peginterferon alfa-2a and weight-based ribavirin for 48 weeks. Patients with a higher viral load and genotype 1 had a lower SVR (47% vs. 65%). For genotype 2 or 3, SVR rates were similar in the four treatment groups (77% to 88%). More severe and serious adverse effects occurred in patients treated for 48 weeks, and patients treated for 48 weeks had higher rates of withdrawal from therapy. Rates of anemia were 3.4%, 10.0%, 6.4%, and 15.4% of patients in groups 24-LD, 24-SD, 48-LD, and 48-SD, respectively. In conclusion, patients with HCV genotype 1 infection should be treated with peginterferon alfa-2a and standard-dose (weight-based) ribavirin for 48 weeks, while patients with HCV genotype 2 or 3 infection may be treated for 24 weeks with peginterferon alfa-2a and lower-dose ribavirin.

Jensen et al, Hepatology, (2006). Early Identification of HCV Genotype 1 Patients Responding to 24 Weeks Peginterferon alfa-2a/Ribavirin Therapy

Study Design

This was a *post hoc* analysis of the phase 3 trial done by Hadziyannis et al. to determine whether patients infected with HCV genotype 1 who achieved an SVR after 24 weeks of treatment could be identified on the basis of RVR at week 4, which was defined as undetectable serum HCV RNA (<50 IU/mL) via qualitative polymerase chain reaction.

Key Findings

Patients with HCV genotype 1 infection who achieved RVR were much more likely to achieve SVR (89% vs. 19%). In addition, in patients with RVR, longer therapy did not improve SVR rates and relapse was uncommon (9%). In those who did not achieve RVR, more intense treatment improved SVR rates, 16% in the group treated for 24 weeks and with low-dose ribavirin compared to 44% in the group treated for 48 weeks and with standard-dose ribavirin. In a multiple logistic regression model, HCV RNA levels were the only independent baseline predictor of RVR (<200,000 IU/mL for subtype 1a and <600,000 IU/mL for subtype 1b). RVR rate is the best predictor of SVR rates, and patients who achieve RVR may be treated for a shorter duration (24 vs. 48 weeks) without a significant effect on SVR rates. In conclusion, in patients with HCV genotype 1 infection, achieving RVR can be used clinically to limit exposure to therapy when the likelihood of response is low, but results need to be confirmed in a prospective trial.

Zeuzem et al, J Hepatology, (2006). Efficacy of 24 weeks treatment with peginterferon alfa-2b plus ribavirin in patients with chronic hepatitis C infected with genotype 1 and low pretreatment viremia

Study Design

This phase 4, open-label, historical-control European study evaluated the safety and efficacy of 24 weeks of treatment with peginterferon alfa-2b 1.5 µg/kg/wk and ribavirin 800 to 1,400 mg/day (weight-based) in treatment-naïve patients with genotype 1 chronic hepatitis C and an HCV-RNA concentration of 600,000 IU/mL or less. The historical-control population was the study population from Manns et al. (2001).

Key Findings

The overall SVR rate was 50% with a predicted response of 69% if data from the study by Manns et al. were used, and therefore 24 weeks of treatment was not as effective as 48 weeks. With multivariable logistic regression analysis, baseline HCV-RNA level and treatment duration of at least 16 weeks were significant predictors of SVR. In addition, undetectable serum HCV-RNA after 4 weeks of therapy (RVR) was an important predictor of SVR, with an SVR rate of 89% for those who achieved RVR versus 25% and 17% for those who had first undetectable HCV-RNA at week 12 or 24, respectively. In addition, a pretreatment HCV-RNA level of 250,000 IU/mL best discriminated between patients with or without SVR after 24 weeks of therapy. Adverse events were noted in 11% of patients, with 3% of patients discontinuing therapy and 26% of patients requiring dose reduction, but these rates were similar to the historical-control study population. In conclusion, 24 weeks of combination therapy with peginterferon alfa-2b and weight-based ribavirin is not as efficacious as 48 weeks for the treatment of patients with genotype 1 chronic hepatitis C with pretreatment HCV-RNA levels of 600,000 IU/mL or less, except in the subset of patients who become undetectable for HCV-RNA at week 4 (RVR).

Jacobson et al, Hepatology, (2007). Peginterferon alfa-2b and weight based or flat-dose ribavirin in chronic hepatitis C patients: a randomized trial (WIN-R trial - Weight-Based Dosing of Peginterferon alfa-2b and Ribavirin)

Study Design

WIN-R was a prospective, multicenter open-label U.S. study to assess whether weight-based dosing (WBD) of peginterferon and ribavirin was superior to flat dosing (FD) as well as to evaluate the efficacy of 24 versus 48 weeks of therapy in patients with genotype 2 or 3 HCV infection.

Key Findings

Patients were more likely to achieve SVR if they received WBD than FD riba-virin, 44.2% versus 40.5% respectively. This was also true in subpopulation anal-ysis—those with genotype 1 infection, African American patients with genotype 1 infection, and patients with genotype 1 infection and baseline viral load above 600,000 IU/mL. In addition, SVR rates decreased as the patient's weight increased in the FD group but were unchanged in the WBD group. For patients with geno-type 2 or 3 infection, treatment for 24 versus 48 weeks provided no additional benefit, 66.2% versus 58.6% respectively. In addition, SVR rates were not differ-ent in the genotype 2 or 3 patients treated for 24 weeks with either WBD or FD. Looking at predictors of response with multivariate regression analysis, ribavirin dosing (WBD vs. FD), genotype (other vs. 1), race (other vs. African American), and cirrhosis (vs. no cirrhosis) were significant predictors of SVR. Finally, adverse events were common, reported by 95% of patients, but were typical of those previously reported for peginterferon and ribavirin therapy. Anemia with hemo-globin below 10 g/dL occurred more often in the WBD group (19.3% vs. 12.5%), but the frequency of other adverse events was similar between the two groups, including significant neutropenia and thrombocytopenia. Discontinuation rates were similar between the two groups. In conclusion, the WIN-R trial confirms that in a large U.S. population, treatment with peginterferon and WBD ribavirin for 48 weeks improves SVR rates for patients with HCV genotype 1 infection, in-cluding a dose of 1,400 mg/d for patients weighing more than 105 kg. In addition, this trial confirmed the equivalent efficacy of 24 versus 48 weeks of combination therapy for patients with HCV genotype 2 or 3 infection.

Di Bisceglie et al, NEJM, (2008). Prolonged therapy of advance chronic hepatitis C with low-dose peginterferon. (HALT-C Trial - Hepatitis C Antiviral Long-Term Treatment against Cirrhosis)

Study Design

HALT-C, a randomized, controlled U.S. trial, compared half-dose peginterferon alfa-2a (90 µg/wk) for 3.5 years versus no therapy for patients with advanced chronic hepatitis C who did not achieve SVR on a previous course of interferon-based therapy without virus eradication. Patients enrolled had advanced hepatic fibrosis on liver biopsy (Ishak fibrosis score of 3 or more) but no history of hepatic decompensation or hepatocellular carcinoma. All patients underwent treatment with peginterferon alfa-2a 180 µg weekly and ribavirin (1,000 to 1,200 mg daily, according to body weight) for at least 24 weeks before undergoing randomization (Fig 15.1).

Key Findings

Patients were followed for primary outcomes including progression of liver disease after randomization—death, hepatic decompensation (variceal hem-orrhage, ascites, spontaneous bacterial peritonitis, or hepatic encephalopathy), hepatocellular carcinoma, Child-Turcotte-Pugh score above 7, or increased

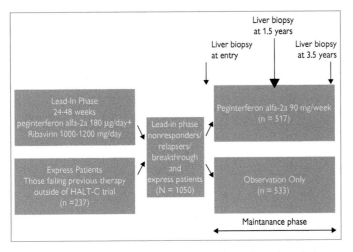

Figure 15.1 Study design for HALT-C Trial, which was designed to evaluate the impact of low-dose peginterferon alfa-2a therapy on the progression of liver fibrosis and clinical outcomes of patients who did not achieve SVR with interferon-based therapy. From CCO: http://www.clinicaloptions.com/Hepatitis/Conference%20Coverage/Milan%20 2008/Tracks/Hepatitis%20C%20Update/Capsules/144.aspx

fibrosis score by 2 or more points on liver biopsy. Treated patients had lower serum ALT levels, with 35% of treated patients with normal ALT compared to 22.6% of untreated patients, and lower HCV RNA levels. Rates of clinical or histologic outcome were similar in the two groups regardless of the presence of cirrhosis at the time of randomization. However, more adverse events were noted in the treatment group, with 32% of patients discontinuing therapy due to anemia, neutropenia, thrombocytopenia, depression, patient refusal, or other reasons. By year 3.5, only 58.9% of patients who were still in the study and had not had a clinical outcome were receiving the full-prescribed dose of peginterferon. In conclusion, long-term maintenance therapy with half-dose peginterferon is ineffective in preventing clinical and histologic disease progression in patients who did not respond to a standard course of peginterferon and ribavirin therapy.

McHutchison et al, NEJM, (2009a). Peginterferon alfa-2b or alfa-2a with ribavirin for treatment of hepatitis C infection (IDEAL Trial - Individualized Dosing Efficacy vs. Flat Dosing to Assess Optimal Pegylated Interferon Therapy)

Study Design

In IDEAL, a randomized, double-blind, U.S. trial, treatment-naïve patients were randomized to three groups: (1) peginterferon alfa-2b 1.5 μg/kg/wk plus ribavirin

800 to 1,400 mg; (2) peginterferon alfa-2b 1.0 μg/kg/wk plus ribavirin 800 to 1,400 mg; (3) peginterferon alfa-2a 180 μg/wk plus ribavirin 800 to 1,200 mg. Treatment groups were also stratified by viral load and race (black vs. non-black). Treatment duration was 48 weeks for all groups.

Key Findings

SVR was not significantly different between the standard-dose peginterferon alfa-2b group (39.8%) versus the low-dose peginterferon alfa-2b group (38%) versus the peginterferon alfa-2a group (40.9%). End-of-treatment responses were higher in the standard-dose peginterferon alfa-2a group, but the relapse rate was also higher. Lower baseline viral load, non-black race, minimal fibrosis, normal baseline fasting glucose, absence of steatosis, and elevated baseline ALT levels were independent predictors of SVR. Increased ribavirin exposure was associated with increased SVR rates. Time to first undetectable HCV RNA was predictive of relapse, with less than 10% of patients who achieved viral clearance by week 4 experiencing relapse compared to 50% of patients clearing virus by week 24. Adverse events and their frequency were similar in the three groups. In conclusion, the rates of SVR and adverse events were similar in patients infected with HCV genotype 1 who received standard-dose or low-dose peginterferon alfa-2b or peginterferon alfa-2a, in combination with ribavirin.

Jensen et al, Ann Intern Med, (2009). Re-treatment of Patients With Chronic Hepatitis C Who Do Not Respond to Peginterferon alfa-2b. (REPEAT Trial— REtreatment with PEgasys® in pATients Not Responding to Prior Peginterferon alfa-2b/ Ribavirin Combination Therapy)

Study Design

REPEAT was a randomized, multicenter trial designed to evaluate the efficacy of retreatment of patients who had not responded to previous treatment with peginterferon alfa-2b plus ribavirin with a 12-week, fixed-dose induction regimen of peginterferon alfa-2a plus standard-dose ribavirin (weight-based dosing) and extended treatment with standard doses of both drugs. Patients were randomized to four groups (Fig. 15.2).

Key Findings

Most of the patients were white (89%) and had genotype 1 infection (91%). While SVR rates in all groups were low with retreatment, patients receiving 72 weeks of therapy were twice as likely to achieve SVR than those receiving 48 weeks of therapy (16% for group A and C vs. 8% for groups B and D). Patients

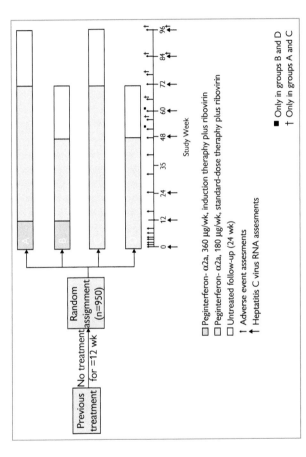

Figure 15.2 Study design for REPEAT Trial, which was designed to evaluate the efficacy of an induction regiment of peginterferon alfa-2a and ribavirin and extended treatment with both drugs. Annals of Internal Medicine 2009 Apr 21;150(8):528–40, with permission from the American College of Physicians.

receiving induction therapy (groups A and B) did not have significantly higher SVR rates than those not receiving induction therapy (groups C and D). EVR rates were higher in the high-dose induction groups (group A and B, 61%, vs. group C and D, 44%), but EVR was not a strong predictor of SVR in this study. Adverse events were similar to those previously reported for patients treated with peginterferon-alfa 2a plus ribavirin and required discontinuation of therapy in a minority of patients (12% in groups A and C, 4% in group B, 6% in group D). Of note, there were significant rates of withdrawal from the study, with about 40% of patients withdrawing from groups A and C versus about 27% from groups B and D. In conclusion, patients who previously did not respond to therapy with peginterferon alfa-2b and ribavirin had very low rates of SVR with retreatment for prolonged durations, with the highest SVR rate for patients retreated for 72 weeks.

Ge et al, Nature, (2009). Genetic variation in IL28B predicts hepatitis C treatment-induced viral clearance.

Study Design

This genome-wide association study (GAWS) was conducted to identify any human genetic contribution to anti-HCV treatment response in patients who were part of the IDEAL study. 1,671 patients were genotyped using Illumina Human610-quad BeadChip and searched for determinants of treatment response, primarily defined as SVR.

Key Findings

Polymorphism on chromosome 19 was strongly associated with SVR in all patients. The location of the polymorphism was 3 kilobases upstream of the *IL28B* gene, which encodes IFN-λ-3. The CC genotype is associated with a two-fold greater SVR rate compared with the TT genotype in patients of European or Hispanic ancestry versus a threefold greater SVR rate in those of African ancestry. Frequency of the C allele also explained about half the difference in SVR rates between patients of European and African ancestry. In addition, from data from a trial of HCV therapy in Asians (Liu et al., 2008), a higher frequency of the C allele was noted in East Asians and was correlated with higher SVR rates in this population compared to those of European and African ancestry. Interestingly, the C allele was associated with a higher baseline viral load, and when compared to ethnically matched controls, the frequency of the C allele was lower in patients with chronic HCV infection. Finally, in a logistic regression model looking at related clinical predictors of SVR rates, the CC genotype was associated with a more substantial difference in SVR rates than other known baseline predictors. In conclusion, advance knowledge of a patient's genotype may identify patients in whom therapy is likely to be successful, and further study into the IFN- λ signaling axis may lead to new potential targets for anti-HCV drug development.

McHutchison et al, NEJM, (2009b). Telaprevir with Peginterferon and Ribavirin for Chronic HCV Genotype 1 Infection (PROVE 1 Trial - Protease Inhibition for Viral Evaluation 1)

Study Design

PROVE 1 was a phase 2, randomized, double-blind, placebo-controlled U.S. trial of telaprevir, a HCV serine protease inhibitor, for patients with genotype 1 HCV infection. The four groups were as follows: (1) The T12PR24 group received telaprevir 750 mg q8h plus peginterferon alfa-2a 180 µg/wk and ribavirin 1,000 to 1,200 mg/day (weight-based) for 12 weeks, followed by peginterferon alfa-2a and ribavirin for 12 more weeks. (2) The T12PR48 group received telaprevir plus peginterferon alfa-2a and ribavirin for 12 weeks, followed by peginterferon alfa-2a and ribavirin for 36 more weeks. (3) The T12PR12 group received telaprevir plus peginterferon alfa-2a and ribavirin for 12 weeks. (4) The PR48 (control) group received placebo plus peginterferon alfa-2a plus ribavirin for 12 weeks followed by peginterferon alfa-2a and ribavirin for 36 more weeks (Fig. 15.3).

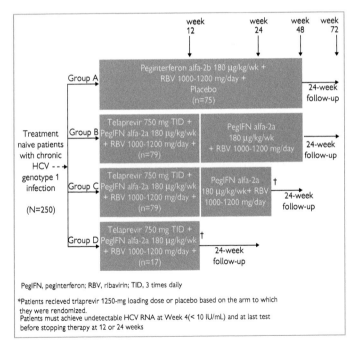

PegIFN, peginterferon; RBV, ribavirin; TID, 3 times daily

*Patients recieved trlaprevir 1250-mg loading dose or placebo based on the arm to which they were rendomized.
Patients must achieve undetectable HCV RNA at Week 4(< 10 IU/mL) and at last test before stopping therapy at 12 or 24 weeks

Figure 15.3 Study design for PROVE 1 Trial, which was designed to evaluate the safety and efficacy of telaprevir in combination with peginterferon alfa-2a and ribavirin in genotype 1 HCV patients.

Key Findings

SVR rates were highest in the T12PR48 group compared to the T12PR24 group versus the PR48 group (67% vs. 61% vs. 41%). Rates of RVR were higher in the T12PR24 and T12PR48 groups compared to the PR48 group. Relapse rates were also lower in the telaprevir-based groups—2% for T12PR24 versus 6% for T12PR48 versus 23% for PR48. The most common adverse events were typical of interferon-based therapy, but rash, pruritus, nausea, and diarrhea were more common in the groups that received telaprevir. Importantly, more patients discontinued therapy in the telaprevir-based groups—21% versus 11% in the PR48 group. Patients receiving telaprevir had 0.5- to 1-g/dL greater decline in hemoglobin at 12 weeks than those in the control group, but this effect was transient. In conclusion, addition of telaprevir significantly increases SVR rates for patients with genotype 1 infection and allows for a shorter duration of therapy (24 vs. 48 weeks) in patients who achieve RVR, with low relapse rates.

Hézode et al, NEJM, (2009). Telaprevir and Peginterferon with or without Ribavirin for Chronic HCV Infection. PROVE 2 Trial

Study Design

PROVE 2 was a phase 2b, randomized, partially double-blind, placebo-controlled European trial to assess the efficacy and adverse-event profile of various regimens combining telaprevir with peginterferon alfa-2a, with or without ribavirin, as compared with peginterferon alfa-2a and ribavirin alone, in treatment-naïve patients infected with HCV genotype 1. (1) The T12PR24 group received telaprevir, peginterferon alfa-2a, and ribavirin for 12 weeks, followed by peginterferon alfa-2a and ribavirin for 12 more weeks. (2) The T12PR12 group received telaprevir, peginterferon alfa-2a, and ribavirin for 12 weeks. (3) The T12P12 group received telaprevir and peginterferon alfa-2a, without ribavirin, for 12 weeks. (4) The PR48 (control) group received placebo, peginterferon alfa-2a, and ribavirin for 12 weeks, followed by peginterferon alfa-2a and ribavirin for 36 more weeks (dosing same as in the PROVE 1 trial, Fig. 15.4).

Key Findings

RVR was achieved more often in the telaprevir-treated groups: 69% of patients in the T12PR24 group, 80% in the T12PR12 group, and 50% in the T12P12 group versus 13% in the PR48 group. EVR rates (at week 12) and end-of-treatment response rates were also higher in the telaprevir-treated groups. SVR rates were higher in the T12PR24 group compared to the PR48 group, 69% versus 46%, but were not significantly different between the T12PR12, T12P12, and PR48 groups (60% vs. 36% vs. 46%). Relapse rates were lower in the T12PR24 group (14%) versus the T12PR12 group (30%) versus the T12P12 group (48%)

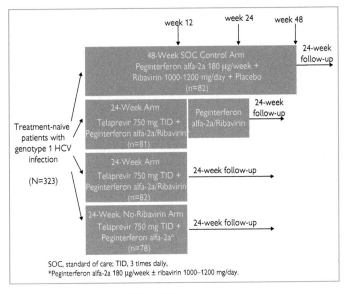

week 12   week 24   week 48

48-Week SOC Control Arm
Peginterferon alfa-2a 180 μg/week +
Ribavirin 1000-1200 mg/day + Placebo
(n=82)

24-week follow-up

Treatment-naive patients with genotype 1 HCV infection

(N=323)

24-Week Arm
Telaprevir 750 mg TID +
Peginterferon alfa-2a/Ribavirin
(n=81)

Peginterferon alfa-2a/Ribavirin

24-week follow-up

24-Week Arm
Telaprevir 750 mg TID +
Peginterferon alfa-2a/Ribavirin
(n=82)

24-week follow-up

24-Week, No-Ribavirin Arm
Telaprevir 750 mg TID +
Peginterferon alfa-2a*
(n=78)

24-week follow-up

SOC, standard of care; TID, 3 times daily,
*Peginterferon alfa-2a 180 μg/week ± ribavirin 1000–1200 mg/day.

Figure 15.4 Study design for PROVE 2 Trial, which was designed to evaluate the efficacy of various regimens of telaprevir with peginterferon alfa-2a with and without ribavirin for the treatment of treatment naïve, genotype 1 HCV patients.

versus the PR group (22%). Treatment group and baseline HCV RNA level were the only two variables significantly associated with SVR. Pruritus and rash were more frequent in the telaprevir groups than in the control group, with about 50% of patients receiving telaprevir experiencing pruritus and rash compared with 35% of patients in the control group. Severe rash occurred in 7% of patients in the T12PR24 group versus 6% in the T12PR12 group versus 3% in the T12P12 group versus 0% in the PR48 group. Anemia was more pronounced in the telaprevir groups, with a median decline of 3.0 g/dL in the PR48 group compared to a 3.6-g/dL decline in the T12PR24 group. In conclusion, adding telaprevir significantly increases SVR rates for patients with genotype 1 infection, and concomitant use of ribavirin is required to achieve the higher SVR rates, largely by preventing relapse and telaprevir resistance.

McHutchison et al, NEJM, (2010). Telaprevir for previously treated Chronic HCV infection. Prove 3 Trial

Study Design

The PROVE 3 trial was a phase 2, randomized, partially placebo-controlled, partially double-blind, international trial. Treatment-experienced patients who had treatment failure (nonresponders and relapsers) were randomized to four groups: (1) the T12PR24 group, receiving telaprevir for 12 weeks and peginterferon alfa-2a (180 µg/wk) and ribavirin (1,000 or 1,200 mg/day, according to body weight) for 24 weeks; (2) the T24PR48 group, receiving telaprevir for 24 weeks and peginterferon alfa-2a and ribavirin for 48 weeks; (3) the T24P24 group, receiving telaprevir and peginterferon alfa-2a for 24 weeks; and (4) the PR48 (or control) group, receiving peginterferon alfa-2a and ribavirin for 48 weeks (Fig. 15.5).

Key Findings

SVR was significantly higher in the three groups receiving telaprevir (51% in the T12PR24 group, 53% in the T24PR48 group, and 24% in the T24P24 group) than in the PR48 group (14%). SVR rates were higher in patients who had relapse versus those who were nonresponders. Relapse rates were lowest in the T24PR48 group (13%) versus the T12PR24 group (30%) versus the T24P24 group (53%) versus the PR48 group (53%). Incidence and severity of rash and pruritus were higher in groups receiving telaprevir, with 5% of patients discontinuing treatment because of rash in the telaprevir groups compared to 0% in the PR48 group. In addition, patients in the telaprevir group were more likely to discontinue therapy due to an adverse event than the PR48 group. In conclusion, telaprevir improves retreatment SVR, but ribavirin should be included in combination therapy with telaprevir and peginterferon alfa-2a. The T12PR24

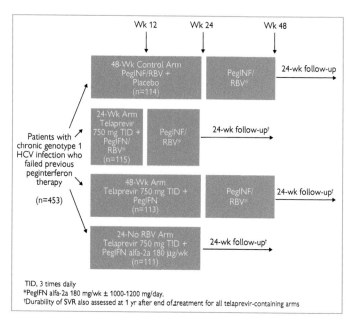

TID, 3 times daily
*PegIFN alfa-2a 180 mg/wk ± 1000-1200 mg/day.
†Durability of SVR also assessed at 1 yr after end of treatment for all telaprevir-containing arms

Figure 15.5 Study design for PROVE 3 Trial, which was designed to evaluate the efficacy of various regimens of telaprevir with peginterferon alfa-2a with and without ribavirin in treatment-experienced, genotype 1 HCV patients.

group had the best risk–benefit profile for treatment, with similar efficacy rates but improved safety and lower discontinuation rates.

Jacobson et al, NEJM, (2011). Telaprevir for Previously Untreated Chronic Hepatitis C Virus Infection. ADVANCE (A new Direction in HCV care: A study of treatment-Naive hepatitis C patients with telaprEvir) Trial

The ADVANCE trial was a phase 3, randomized, double-blind, placebo-controlled international trial for telaprevir for patients with previously untreated chronic hepatitis C. Patients were randomized to three groups: (1) T12PR group, receiving telaprevir for 12 weeks and peginterferon alfa-2a (180 μg/wk) and ribavirin (1,000 or 1,200 mg/d, according to body weight) for 24 to 48 weeks; (2) the T8PR group, receiving telaprevir for 8 weeks and peginterferon alfa-2a and ribavirin for 24-48 weeks; (3) the PR48 (or control) group, receiving placebo for 12 weeks and peginterferon alfa-2a and ribavirin for 48 weeks (Fig. 15.6).

Key Findings

Patients in the telaprevir group were more likely to achieve SVR, 75% in the T12PR group versus 69% in the T8PR group versus 44% in the PR group. RVR was seen in 68%, 66%, and 9% of the three groups, respectively. Among the patients with extended rapid virologic response assigned to receive a total of 24 weeks of therapy, 89% in the T12PR group and 83% in the T8PR group achieved SVR. Higher SVR rates were also seen in subgroup analysis of patients with genotype 1a versus 1b infection, patients of African American race, patients with baseline viral load above 800,000 IU/mL, and patient with bridging fibrosis or cirrhosis. In addition, relapse occurred in 9% of the T12PR group, 9% of the T8PR group, and 28% of the PR group. Virologic failure rates were higher in the T8PR group (10%) versus the T12PR group (5%) and attributed to emergence of lower-level resistant variants. Adverse events including nausea, diarrhea, pruritus, rash, and anemia occurred more often in the telaprevir groups with higher discontinuation rates (11% in the T12PR group, 7% in the T8PR group, 1% in the PR group), mostly due to rash and anemia. In conclusion, this phase 3 trial confirmed the findings of the PROVE 1 and PROVE 2 trials: telaprevir used for the first 12 weeks of treatment with peginterferon and ribavirin improves SVR rates in patients with genotype 1 chronic hepatitis C and allows for shortening therapy to 24 weeks for patients achieving RVR and EVR.

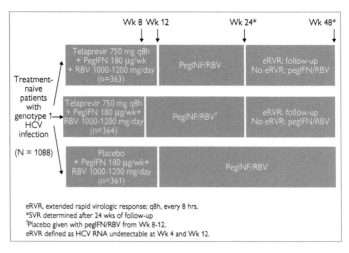

Figure 15.6 Study design for ADVANCE Trial, which was designed to evaluate the efficacy of 12 vs. 8 weeks of telaprevir in combination with peginterferon alfa-2a with ribavirin for 24 vs. 48 weeks depending on early viral kinetics for treatment naïve genotype 1 HCV patients.

Sherman et al, NEJM, (2011). **Response-Guided Telaprevir combination treatment for hepatitis C virus infection. ILLUMINATE (ILLUstrating the Effects of CoMbINAtion Therapy with TElaprevir) Trial**

Study Design

ILLUMINATE was a phase 3, open-label, randomized, non-inferiority international trial to assess the non-inferiority of a 24-week versus a 48-week telaprevir-based regimen for patients with extended rapid virologic response (extended RVR; undetectable HCV RNA levels at weeks 4 and 12). All patients received telaprevir at a dose of 750 mg every 8 hours, peginterferon alfa-2a at a dose of 180 µg per week, and ribavirin at a dose of 1,000 to 1,200 mg per day, for 12 weeks. Patients with an extended RVR were randomized at week 20 to receive peginterferon–ribavirin for either an additional 12 weeks (T12PR24) or 36 weeks (T12PR48). Patients without an extended RVR were assigned to T12PR48 (Fig. 15.7).

Key Findings

Most of the patients were white, 28% had bridging fibrosis or cirrhosis, and 72% had genotype subtype 1a infection. A majority of the study patients (72%) achieved RVR at week 4; 65% achieved extended RVR. While the overall SVR rate was 72%, of the patients achieving extended RVR, 92% of those assigned

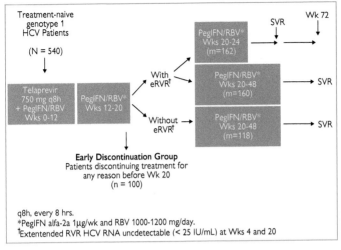

q8h, every 8 hrs.
*PegIFN alfa-2a 1μg/wk and RBV 1000-1200 mg/day.
†Extentended RVR HCV RNA uncdetectable (< 25 IU/mL) at Wks 4 and 20

Figure 15.7 Study design for ILLUMINATE Trial, which was designed to evaluate the non-inferiority of 24 vs. 48-week telaprevir-based regimen for patients with extended RVR.

to the T12PR24 group achieved SVR and 88% of those assigned to T12PR48 group achieved SVR. More patients in the T12PR24 group completed therapy compared to the T12PR48 group (99% vs. 74%). Of the patients who did not achieve extended RVR and who were assigned to the T12PR48 group, 64% achieved SVR. 100 patients (18.5%) discontinued therapy before week 20, and the SVR rate was 23% in this group. The relapse rates in the groups were also low and similar: 6% in the T12PR24 group, 3% in the T12PR48 group, 11% in the T12PR48 group who did not achieve extended RVR. A shorter duration of therapy did not adversely affect the SVR rates in historically hard-to-treat groups of patients such as those with high viral load, those with genotype subtype 1a versus 1b infection, those with bridging fibrosis or cirrhosis, and white versus black patients. Overall, 9% of patients had serious adverse events, with anemia being the most common. Adverse events were more common in the T12PR48 group compared to the T12PR24 group (10% vs. 2%). During the telaprevir treatment phase, 7% of patients discontinued all study drugs, with 1% due to rash and 1% due to anemia. The ribavirin dose was modified in 46% of patients due to anemia. In conclusion, response-guided therapy for 24 weeks was non-inferior to 48 weeks for treatment-naïve patients with genotype subtype 1a HCV infection who achieved extended RVR, even in patients who are historically difficult to treat. In addition, fewer adverse events and treatment discontinuations were seen in patients treated for a shorter period of time.

Zeuzem et al, NEJM, (2011). Telaprevir for Retreatment of HCV Infection. REALIZE (REtreAtment of nonresponders to peginferon/ribavirin with teLaprevir based regimen to optimIZE outcomes) Trial

Study Design

REALIZE was a phase 3, randomized, double-blind, placebo-controlled trial to evaluate the efficacy and safety of retreatment of patients with chronic HCV genotype 1 infection with telaprevir in combination with peginterferon and riba-virin. Patients included were nonresponders, partial responders, and relapsers and were randomly assigned to three groups: (1) the T12PR48 group, receiving telaprevir 750 mg q8h, peginterferon alfa-2a (180 µg/wk), and ribavirin (1,000 or 1,200 mg/day, according to body weight) for 12 weeks, followed by placebo plus peginterferon and ribavirin for 4 weeks, and then peginterferon plus ri-bavirin alone for 32 weeks; (2) the lead-in T12PR48 group, receiving placebo, peginterferon, and ribavirin for 4 weeks, followed by telaprevir for 12 weeks and peginterferon alfa-2a and ribavirin for 32 weeks; (3) the PR48 (control) group, receiving placebo, peginterferon alfa-2a, and ribavirin for 16 weeks fol-lowed by peginterferon and ribavirin for 32 weeks (Fig. 15.8).

Key Findings

Previous treatment had resulted in relapse in 53% of patients, partial response in 19%, and no response in 19%. SVR rates were significantly higher in groups

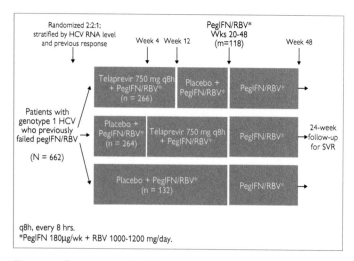

q8h, every 8 hrs.
*PeglFN 180µg/wk + RBV 1000-1200 mg/day.

Figure 15.8 Study design for REALIZE Trial, which was designed to evaluate the safety and efficacy of retreatment of genotype 1 HCV patients with telaprevir in combination with peginterferon alfa-2a and ribavirin.

receiving telaprevir. For prior relapsers, SVR rates were 83% in the T12PR48 group,

88% in the lead-in T12PR48 group, and 24% in the control group. For patients with prior partial response, SVR rates were 59% in the T12PR48 group, 54% in the lead-in T12PR48 group, and 15% in the control group. For prior nonresponders, SVR rates were 29% in the T12PR48 group, 33% in the lead-in T12PR48 group, and 5% in the control group. There was no statistical difference between the SVR rates for the T12PR48 versus lead-in T12PR48 groups in each of the three subgroups of patients. Relapse rates were lower in the two telaprevir groups, and 73% of these were associated with telaprevir resistance. Adverse events were more frequent in the two telaprevir groups, with fatigue, pruritus, rash, nausea, influenza-like illness, anemia, and diarrhea occurring most frequently. Serious adverse events leading to discontinuation of therapy in the telaprevir groups occurred in 13% of patients compared with 3% in the control group, with 5% of patients stopping telaprevir therapy due to a skin event. In conclusion, adding telaprevir to peginterferon and ribavirin greatly improves SVR rates for patients with chronic HCV genotype 1 infection who previously did not achieve SVR with peginterferon and ribavirin alone, but lead-in therapy with peginterferon and ribavirin did not improve the efficacy of triple therapy.

Kwo et al, Lancet, (2010). **Efficacy of boceprevir, an NS3 protease inhibitor, in combination with peginterferon alfa-2b and ribavirin in treatment-naive patients with genotype 1 hepatitis C infection: an open-label, randomised, multicentre phase 2 trial. SPRINT-1 Trial [SPRINT-1 (Serine Protease Inhibitor Therapy-1) study]**

Study Design

SPRINT 1 was a phase 2 international trial of boceprevir, a direct-acting serine protease inhibitor, evaluating its safety and efficacy when used in combination with peginterferon and ribavirin in a variety of different dosing combinations (Fig. 15.9) for patients with chronic hepatitis C due to genotype 1 infection: (1) PR4 (lead-in): peginterferon alfa-2b 1.5 μg/kg plus ribavirin 800 to 1,400 mg/day for 4 weeks; (2) PR48 (control): peginterferon alfa-2b 1.5 μg/kg plus ribavirin 800 to 1,400 mg/day for 48 weeks; (3) PRB24/28/44/48: peginterferon alfa-2b, ribavirin, and boceprevir 800 mg three times a day for 24, 28, 44, or 48 weeks; (4) Low-dose PRB48: peginterferon alfa-2b, ribavirin 400 to 1,000 mg, and boceprevir 800 mg three times a day for 48 weeks. Patients in all groups were followed up for 24 weeks after the end of treatment.

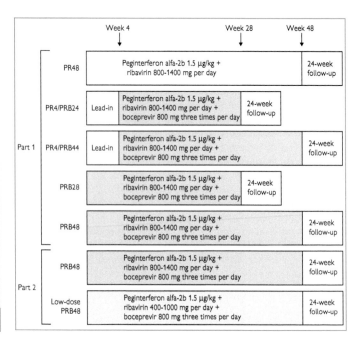

Figure 15.9 Study design of SPRINT-1 Trial, which was designed to evaluate the safety and efficacy of boceprevir when used in combination with peg-interferon alfa-2b and ribavirin in various treatment regimens.

Key Findings

SVR rates in the four boceprevir groups were higher than in the PR48 control group—56% in the PR4/PRB24 group, 54% in the PRB28 group, 75% in the PR4/PRB44 group, 67% in the PRB48 group, 36% in the low-dose PRB48 group, 39% in the PR48 (control) group. Relapse rates were lower in the 48-week treatment groups receiving boceprevir. The low-dose PRB therapy was associated with high relapse rates. RVR was highly predictive of SVR: of the patients who achieved RVR, 82% of the PR4/PRB24 group, 74% of the PRB28 group, 94% of the PR4/PRB44 group, and 84% of the PRB48 group also achieved SVR. Comparing those in the lead-in versus no lead-in groups, higher SVR was noted in participants with less than 1.5 $\log_{10}$ reduction from baseline at week 4 who received PRB for 44 weeks. The most common adverse events reported in the boceprevir group were fatigue, anemia, nausea, and headache, similar to the group not receiving boceprevir. Anemia was more frequent in the boceprevir group, but dose reduction of ribavirin was similar between all groups. Treatment discontinuation related to adverse events was more frequent in the boceprevir group, ranging from 9% to 19% versus 8% in the control group. In conclusion, boceprevir significantly increases the chances of SVR when combined with peginterferon and ribavirin, especially if 48 weeks of therapy are completed and a lead-in phase is used.

Poordad et al, NEJM, (2011). Boceprevir for untreated chronic HCV genotype 1 infection. SPRINT-2 Trial

Study Design

SPRINT 2 was a phase 3, international, randomized, blinded, placebo-controlled trial to evaluate the safety and efficacy of boceprevir in combination with peginterferon and ribavirin after a lead-in period in black and non-black patients. Treatment groups are shown in Figure 15.10. Peginterferon alfa-2b 1.5 µg/kg/wk, ribavirin 600 to 1,400 mg/day, and boceprevir 800 mg three times daily were used. Non-black patients and black patients were recruited and randomized separately.

Key Findings

SVR rates were significantly higher in the groups receiving boceprevir, both in the non-black and black cohort. In the non-black cohort, SVR rates were 67% in group 2, 68% in group 3, and 40% in group 1 (control). In the black cohort, SVR rates were 23% in group 1, 42% in group 2, and 53% in group 3. The SVR rate for patients whose HCV RNA level became undetectable by week 8 and stayed undetectable through week 24 was 97% in group 2 and 96% in group 3 for the non-black cohort. Relapse rates were also lower in the two boceprevir groups. The most frequent adverse events were fatigue, headache, and nausea. Dysguesia and anemia occurred more often in the boceprevir-treated groups, with 13% of controls and 21% of boceprevir recipients requiring dose reductions because of anemia. In conclusion, adding boceprevir to peginterferon and ribavirin significantly improves SVR rates for both black and non-black patients, even if patients do not achieve a decrease of more than 1 $\log_{10}$ at week 4. In

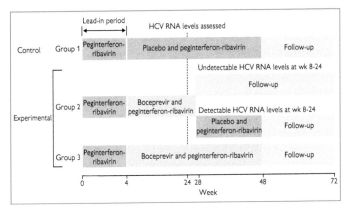

Figure 15.10 Study design for SPRINT-2 Trial, which was designed to evaluate the efficacy of response guided treatment with boceprevir, peginterferon alfa-2b, and ribavirin after a lead-in period in 2 cohorts, black and non-black patients. The New England Journal of Medicine 2011 Mar 31;364(13):1195–206, with permission from the Massachusetts Medical Society.

addition, therapy guided to response at 24 weeks resulted in SVR rates that were similar in patients treated for 24 versus 44 weeks.

> ## Bacon et al, NEJM, (2011). Boceprevir for previously treated chronic HCV genotype 1 infection. Retreatment with HCV Serine Protease Inhibitor Boceprevir and PegIntron/Rebetol 2 (RESPOND-2—Retreatment with HCV Serine Protease Inhibitor Boceprevir and PegIntron/Rebetol 2)

Study Design

RESPOND 2 was a phase 3, international, randomized, double-blind, place-bo-controlled trial to evaluate the safety and efficacy of boceprevir in combination with peginterferon and ribavirin for patients whose HCV genotype 1 infection previously did not respond to peginterferon and ribavirin therapy. Peginterferon alfa-2b 1.5 µg/kg/wk, ribavirin 600 to 1,400 mg/day, and boceprevir 800 mg three times daily were used. Randomized patients were stratified by previous response (nonresponse vs. relapse) and HCV sub-genotype (1a vs. 1b) (Fig. 15.11).

Key Findings

SVR rates were significantly higher for patients receiving boceprevir: 21% in group 1, 59% in group 2, 66% in group 3. In relapsers, SVR rates were 29% in group 1, 69% in group 2, and 75% in group 3, while in nonresponders, SVR rates were 7%, 40%, and 52% in groups 1, 2, and 3, respectively. Patients who were labeled "interferon responders" (decrease in HCV RNA level 1 $\log_{10}$ IU/mL or more after 4 week lead-in period) had much higher SVR rates in all three groups: 0% versus 25%, 33% versus 73%, and 34% versus 79% in groups 1, 2, and 3, respectively. The odds of a SVR was greater, across all subgroups, with either response-guided triple therapy (group 2) or 44-week triple therapy (group 3) than with the standard of care (group 1). Baseline factors associated with improved SVR rates included assignment to boceprevir group, previous relapse versus nonresponse, low viral load at baseline, and absence of cirrhosis, but sub-genotype was not important. Importantly, 61% of patients in group 1 discontinued therapy at week 12 due to the predefined stopping rule versus only 22% and 18% of patients in groups 2 and 3, respectively, meaning that treatment durations were significantly longer in the boceprevir groups. The most common adverse events were influenza-like symptoms. There was a higher incidence of anemia in the boceprevir groups, and there were more discontinuations and dose modifications owing to adverse events in the boceprevir groups. In conclusion, adding boceprevir to peginterferon and ribavirin significantly increases SVR rates for patients undergoing retreatment for genotype 1 HCV infection, even if patients have a poor response to interferon during the lead-in period.

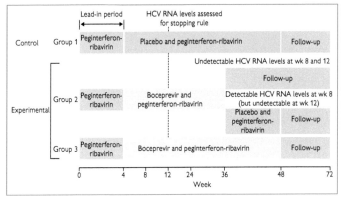

Figure 15.11 Study design for RESPOND-2 Trial, which was designed to evaluate the safety and efficacy of response guided therapy with boceprevir, peginterferon and ribavirin for treatment-experienced patients genotype 1 HCV patients.

Gane et al, Lancet, (2010). **Oral combination therapy with a nucleoside polymerase inhibitor (RG7128) and danoprevir for chronic hepatitis C genotype 1 infection: a randomised, double-blind, placebo-controlled, dose-escalation trial. INFORM-1 (INterferon-Free regimen fOR the Management of HCV) Trial.**

Study Design

INFORM 1 was a phase 1, randomized, double-blind, placebo-controlled, dose-escalation trial in New Zealand and Australia enrolling patients with HCV genotype 1 infection without cirrhosis, with normal renal and hepatic function, and without clinically significant cardiovascular or cerebrovascular disease. Patients were treatment-naïve or treatment-experienced (null responders, partial responders, or relapsers). Patients were assigned to one of seven cohorts and then randomly assigned to treatment or placebo. The primary outcome was change in HCV RNA concentration from baseline to day 14 in patients who received 13 days of combination treatment.

Key Findings

Most of the patients were white (90%) and male (80%) and had genotype 1a infection (70%). Median reduction in HCV RNA concentrations were about 5 $\log_{10}$ IU/mL, with similar response rates between genotype 1a and 1b patients. Of the patients in the highest-dose groups, cohorts F and G, 5/8 (62.5%) of treatment-naïve patients and 2/8 (25%) of null responders had undetectable HCV RNA concentrations at day 14. No evidence of treatment-emergent resistance was identified. The combination of RG7128 and danoprevir was well tolerated, with the most common adverse event being headache, which occurred in 13% to 88% of the treatment cohorts versus 57% in the placebo group. Other common adverse events were lethargy, rash, gastrointestinal disorders, and nausea. There were no treatment withdrawals or dose reductions. In conclusion, the study confirms the safety of combination oral direct-acting antiviral drugs without pegylated interferon and provides proof of concept for an interferon, oral approach to the treatment of chronic hepatitis C.

References

Bacon, B. R., S. C. Gordon, E. Lawitz, et al. (2011). Boceprevir for previously treated chronic HCV genotype 1 infection. *New England Journal of Medicine, 364,* 1207–1217.

Davis, G. L., L. A. Balart, E. R. Schiff, et al. (1989). Treatment of chronic hepatitis C with recombinant interferon alfa. A multicenter randomized, controlled trial. Hepatitis Interventional Therapy Group. *New England Journal of Medicine, 321,* 1501–1506.

Di Bisceglie, A. M., M. L. Shiffman, G. T. Everson, et al. (2008). Prolonged therapy of advanced chronic hepatitis C with low-dose peginterferon. *New England Journal of Medicine, 359,* 2429–2441.

Fried, M. W., M. L. Shiffman, K. R. Reddy, et al. (2002). Peginterferon alfa-2a plus ribavirin for chronic hepatitis C virus infection. *New England Journal of Medicine, 347,* 975–982.

Gane, E. J., S. K. Roberts, C. A. Stedman, et al. (2010). Oral combination therapy with a nucleoside polymerase inhibitor (RG7128) and danoprevir for chronic hepatitis C genotype 1 infection (INFORM-1): a randomised, double-blind, placebo-controlled, dose-escalation trial. *Lancet, 376,* 1467–1475.

Ge, D., J. Fellay, A. J. Thompson, et al. (2009). Genetic variation in IL28B predicts hepatitis C treatment-induced viral clearance. *Nature, 461,* 399–401.

Hadziyannis, S. J., H. Sette Jr., T. R. Morgan, et al. (2004). Peginterferon-alpha2a and ribavirin combination therapy in chronic hepatitis C: a randomized study of treatment duration and ribavirin dose. *Annals of Internal Medicine, 140,* 346–355.

Hézode, C., N. Forestier, G. Dusheiko, et al. (2009). Telaprevir and peginterferon with or without ribavirin for chronic HCV infection. *New England Journal of Medicine, 360,* 1839–1850.

Hoofnagle, J. H., K. D. Mullen, D. B. Jones, et al. (1986). Treatment of chronic non-A, non-B hepatitis with recombinant human alpha interferon. A preliminary report. *New England Journal of Medicine, 315,* 1575–1578.

Jacobson, I. M., R. S. Brown Jr., B. Freilich B, et al. (2007). Peginterferon alfa-2b and weight-based or flat-dose ribavirin in chronic hepatitis C patients: a randomized trial. *Hepatology, 46,* 971–981.

Jacobson, I. M., J. G. McHutchison, G. Dusheiko, et al. (2011). Telaprevir for previously untreated chronic hepatitis C virus infection. *New England Journal of Medicine, 364,* 2405–2416.

Jensen, D. M., T. R. Morgan, P. Marcellin, et al. (2006). Early identification of HCV ge-notype 1 patients responding to 24 weeks peginterferon alpha-2a (40 kd)/ribavirin therapy. *Hepatology, 43,* 954–960.

Jensen, D. M., P. Marcellin, B. Freilich, et al. (2009). Re-treatment of patients with chronic hepatitis C who do not respond to peginterferon-alpha2b: a randomized trial. *Annals of Internal Medicine, 150,* 528–540.

Kwo, P. Y., E. J. Lawitz, J. McCone, et al. (2010). Efficacy of boceprevir, an NS3 prote-ase inhibitor, in combination with peginterferon alfa-2b and ribavirin in treatment-naive patients with genotype 1 hepatitis C infection (SPRINT-1): an open-label, randomised, multicentre phase 2 trial. *Lancet, 376,* 705–716.

Lai, M. Y., J. H. Kao, P. M. Yang, et al. (1996). Long-term efficacy of ribavirin plus interferon alfa in the treatment of chronic hepatitis C. *Gastroenterology, 111,* 1307–1312.

Liu, C. H., C. J. Liu, C. L. Lin CL, et al. (2008). Pegylated interferon-alpha-2a plus riba-virin for treatment-naive Asian patients with hepatitis C virus genotype 1 infec-tion: a multicenter, randomized controlled trial. *Clinical Infectious Diseases, 47,* 1260–1269.

Manns, M. P., J. G. McHutchison, S. C. Gordon, et al. (2001). Peginterferon alfa-2b plus ribavirin compared with interferon alfa-2b plus ribavirin for initial treatment of chronic hepatitis C: a randomised trial. *Lancet, 358,* 958–965.

McHutchison, J. G., S. C. Gordon, E. R. Schiff, et al. (1998). Interferon alfa-2b alone or in combination with ribavirin as initial treatment for chronic hepatitis C. Hepatitis Interventional Therapy Group. *New England Journal of Medicine, 339,* 1485–1492.

McHutchison, J. G., E. J. Lawitz, M. L. Shiffman, et al. (2009a). Peginterferon alfa-2b or alfa-2a with ribavirin for treatment of hepatitis C infection. *New England Journal of Medicine, 361,* 580–593.

McHutchison, J. G., G. T. Everson, S. C. Gordon, et al. (2009b). Telaprevir with peginterferon and ribavirin for chronic HCV genotype 1 infection. *New England Journal of Medicine, 360,* 1827–1838.

McHutchison, J. G., M. P. Manns, A. J. Muir, et al. (2010). Telaprevir for previ-ously treated chronic HCV infection. *New England Journal of Medicine, 362,* 1292–1303.

Poordad, F., J. McCone Jr., B. R. Bacon, et al. (2011). Boceprevir for untreated chronic HCV genotype 1 infection. *New England Journal of Medicine, 364,* 1195–1206.

Sherman, K. E., S. L. Flamm, N. H. Afdhal, et al. (2011). Response-guided telaprevir combination treatment for hepatitis C virus infection. *New England Journal of Medicine, 365,* 1014–1024.

Zeuzem, S., S. V. Feinman, J. Rasenack, et al. (2000). Peginterferon alfa-2a in patients with chronic hepatitis C. *New England Journal of Medicine, 343,* 1666–1672.

Zeuzem, S., M. Buti, P. Ferenci, et al. (2006). Efficacy of 24 weeks treatment with peginterferon alfa-2b plus ribavirin in patients with chronic hepatitis C infected with genotype 1 and low pretreatment viremia. *Journal of Hepatology, 44,* 97–103.

Zeuzem, S., P. Andreone, S. Pol, et al. (2011). Telaprevir for retreatment of HCV infection. *New England Journal of Medicine, 364,* 2417–2428.

Appendix

Table 1 Drugs that Are Contraindicated with INCIVEK		
Drug	**Class DrugsWithin Class that are Contraindicated with INCIVEK**	**Clinical Comments**
Alpha 1adrenoreceptor antagonist	Alfuzosin	Potential for hypotension or cardiac arrhythmia
Antimycobacterials	Rifampin	Rifampin significantly reduces telaprevir plasma concentrations.
Ergot derivatives	Dihydroergotamine, ergonovine, ergotamine, methylergonovine	Potential for acute ergot toxicity characterized by peripheral vasospasm or ischemia
GI motility agent	Cisapride	Potential for cardiac arrhythmias
Herbal products	St. John's wort (*Hypericum perforatum*)	Plasma concentrations of telaprevir can be reducedby concomitant use of the herbal preparation St.John's wort.
HMG CoA reductase inhibitors	Lovastatin, simvastatin	Potential for myopathy, including rhabdomyolysis
Neuroleptic	Pimozide	Potential for serious and/or life-threatening adverse reactions such as cardiac arrhythmias secondary to increases in plasma concentrations of antiarrhythmics
PDE5 inhibitor	Sildenafil (Revatio®) or tadalafil (Adcirca®) (for treatment of pulmonary arterial hypertension)	Potential for PDE5 inhibitor-associated adverse events, including visual abnormalities, hypotension, prolonged erection, and syncope
Sedatives/hypnotics	Orally administered midazolam, triazolam	Prolonged or increased sedation or respiratory depression

©2011 Vertex Pharmaceuticals Incorporated.

Table 2 Clinical Adverse Drug Reactions Reported with at Least 5% Higher Frequency Among Subjects Receiving INCIVEK

	INCIVEK, Peginterferon alfa, and Ribavirin Combination Treatment (N=1,797)	Peginterferon alfa and Ribavirin (N=493)
Rash*	56%	34%
Fatigue	56%	50%
Pruritus	47%	28%
Nausea	39%	28%
Anemia*	36%	17%
Diarrhea	26%	17%
Vomiting	13%	8%
Hemorrhoids	12%	3%
Anorectal discomfort	11%	3%
Dysgeusia	10%	3%
Anal pruritus	6%	1%

* Rash and anemia based on SSC (Special Search Category) grouped terms.

Table 3

Concomitant Drug Class: Drug Name	Effect on Concentration of INCIVEK or Concomitant Drug	Clinical Comment
ANTIARRHYTHMICS		
lidocaine (systemic), amiodarone, bepridil, flecainide, propafenone, quinidine	↓ antiarrhythmics	Co-administration with telaprevir has the potential to produce serious and/or life-threatening adverse events and has not been studied. Caution is warranted and clinical monitoring is recommended when coadministered with telaprevir.
digoxin*	↓ digoxin	Concentrations of digoxin were increased when co-administered with telaprevir. The lowest dose of digoxin should be initially prescribed. The serum digoxin concentrations should be monitored and used for titration of digoxin dose to obtain the desired clinical effect.
ANTIBACTERIALS		
clarithromycin erythromycin telithromycin	↓ telaprevir ↓ antibacterials	Concentrations of both telaprevir and the antibacterial may be increased during co-administration. Caution is warranted and clinical monitoring is recommended when co-administered with telaprevir. QT interval prolongation and torsade de Pointes have been reported with clarithromycin and erythromycin. QT interval prolongation has been reported with telithromycin.
ANTICOAGULANT		
warfarin	↓ or ↑ warfarin	Concentrations of warfarin may be altered when co-administered with telaprevir. The international normalized ratio (INR) should be monitored when warfarin is co-administered with telaprevir.

(continued)

Table 3 Continued

Concomitant Drug Class: Drug Name	Effect on Concentration of INCIVEK or Concomitant Drug	Clinical Comment
ANTICONVULSANTS		
carbamazepine phenobarbital phenytoin	↑ telaprevir ↓carbamazepine ↓ or ↑ phenytoin ↓ or ↑ phenobarbital	Concentrations of the anticonvulsant may be altered and concentrations of telaprevir may be decreased. Caution should be used when prescribing carbamazepine, phenobarbital, and phenytoin. Telaprevir may be less effective in patients taking these agents concomitantly. Clinical or laboratory monitoring of carbamazepine, phenobarbital, and phenytoin concentrations and dose titration are recommended to achieve the desired clinical response.
ANTIDEPRESSANTS		
escitalopram* desipramine trazodone	↔ telaprevir ↑ escitalopram ↓ desipramine ↓ trazodone	Concentrations of escitalopram were decreased when co-administered with telaprevir. Selective serotonin reuptake inhibitors such as escitalopram have a wide therapeutic index, but doses may need to be adjusted when combined with telaprevir. Concomitant use of trazodone or desipramine and telaprevir may increase plasma concentrations of trazodone or desipramine, which may lead to adverse events such as nausea, dizziness, hypotension, and syncope. If trazodone or desipramine is used with telaprevir, the combination should be used with caution and a lower dose of trazodone or desipramine should be considered.

ANTIFUNGALS		
ketoconazole* itraconazole posaconazole voriconazole	↓ ketoconazole ↓telaprevir ↓ itraconazole ↓ posaconazole ↓ or ↑ voriconazole	Ketoconazole increases the plasma concentrations of telaprevir. Concomitant systemic use of itraconazole or posaconazole with telaprevir may increase the plasma concentration of telaprevir. Plasma concentrations of itraconazole, ketoconazole, or posaconazole may be increased in the presence of telaprevir. When co-administration is required, high doses of itraconazole or ketoconazole (greater than 200 mg/day) are not recommended. Caution is warranted and clinical monitoring is recommended for itraconazole, posaconazole, and voriconazole. QT interval prolongation and torsade de Pointes have been reported with voriconazole and posaconazole. QT interval prolongation has been reported with ketoconazole. Due to multiple enzymes involved with voriconazole metabolism, it is difficult to predict the interaction with telaprevir. Voriconazole should not be administered to patients receiving telaprevir unless an assessment of the benefit/risk ratio justifies its use.
ANTI-GOUT		
colchicine	↓ colchicine	Patients with renal or hepatic impairment should not be given colchicine with telaprevir, due to the risk of colchicine toxicity. A reduction in colchicine dosage or an interruption of colchicine treatment is recommended in patients with normal renal or hepatic function. Treatment of gout flares: co-administration of colchicine in patients on telaprevir: 0.6 mg (1 tablet) for 1 dose, followed by 0.3 mg (half tablet) 1 hour later. Not to be repeated before 3 days. If used for prophylaxis of gout flares: co-administration of colchicine in patients on telaprevir: If the original regimen was 0.6 mg twice a day, the regimen should be adjusted to 0.3 mg once a day. If the original regimen was 0.6 mg once a day, the regimen should be adjusted to 0.3 mg once every other day. Treatment of familial Mediterranean fever (FMF): co-administration of colchicine in patients on telaprevir: Maximum daily dose of 0.6 mg (may be given as 0.3 mg twice a day).

(continued)

Table 3 Continued

Concomitant Drug Class: Drug Name	Effect on Concentration of INCIVEK or Concomitant Drug	Clinical Comment
ANTIMYCOBACTERIAL		
rifabutin	↑ telaprevir ↓ rifabutin	Concentrations of telaprevir may be decreased, while rifabutin concentrations may be increased during coadministration. Telaprevir may be less effective due to decreased concentrations. The concomitant use of rifabutin and telaprevir is not recommended.
BENZODIAZEPINES		
alprazolam*	↓ alprazolam	Concomitant use of alprazolam and telaprevir increases exposure to alprazolam. Clinical monitoring is warranted.
parenterally administered midazolam*	↓ midazolam	Concomitant use of parenterally administered midazolam with telaprevir increased exposure to midazolam. Co-administration should be done in a setting that ensures clinical monitoring and appropriate medical management in case of respiratory depression and/or prolonged sedation. Dose reduction for midazolam should be considered, especially if more than a single dose of midazolam is administered. Co-administration of oral midazolam with telaprevir is contraindicated.
zolpidem (nonbenzodiazepine sedative)*	↑ zolpidem	Exposure to zolpidem was decreased when co-administered with telaprevir. Clinical monitoring and dose titration of zolpidem is recommended to achieve the desired clinical response.
CALCIUM CHANNEL BLOCKERS		
amlodipine* diltiazem felodipine nicardipine nifedipine nisoldipine verapamil	↓ amlodipine ↓ calcium channel blockers	Exposure to amlodipine was increased when co-administered with telaprevir. Caution should be used and dose reduction for amlodipine should be considered. Clinical monitoring of other calcium channel blockers may be increased when telaprevir is co-administered. Caution is warranted and clinical monitoring of patients is recommended.

CORTICOSTEROIDS		
Systemic prednisone methylprednisolone	↓prednisone ↓methylprednisolone	Systemic corticosteroids such as prednisone and methylprednisolone are CYP3A substrates. Since telaprevir is a potent CYP3A inhibitor, plasma concentrations of these corticosteroids can be increased significantly. Co-administration of systemic corticosteroids and telaprevir is not recommended [see *Warnings and Precautions (5.3)*].
Systemic dexamethasone	↑ telaprevir	Systemic dexamethasone induces CYP3A and can thereby decrease telaprevir plasma concentrations. This may result in loss of therapeutic effect of telaprevir. Therefore, this combination should be used with caution or alternatives should be considered.
Inhaled/Nasal fluticasone budesonide	↓ fluticasone ↓ budesonide	Concomitant use of inhaled fluticasone or budesonide and telaprevir may increase plasma concentrations of fluticasone or budesonide, resulting in significantly reduced serum cortisol concentrations. Co-administration of fluticasone or budesonide and telaprevir is not recommended unless the potential benefit to the patient outweighs the risk of systemic corticosteroid side effects.
ENDOTHELIN RECEPTOR ANTAGONIST		
bosentan	↓ bosentan	Concentrations of bosentan may be increased when co-administered with telaprevir. Caution is warranted and clinical monitoring is recommended.
HIV-ANTIVIRAL AGENTS: HIV-PROTEASE INHIBITORS (PIs)		
atazanavir/ritonavir*	↑ telaprevir ↓ atazanavir	Concomitant administration of telaprevir and atazanavir/ritonavir resulted in reduced steady-state telaprevir exposure, while steady-state atazanavir exposure was increased.
darunavir/ritonavir*	↑ telaprevir ↑darunavir	Concomitant administration of telaprevir and darunavir/ritonavir resulted in reduced steady-state exposures to telaprevir and darunavir. It is not recommended to co-administer darunavir/ritonavir and telaprevir.
fosamprenavir/ritonavir*	↑ telaprevir ↑fosamprenavir	Concomitant administration of telaprevir and fosamprenavir/ritonavir resulted in reduced steady-state exposures to telaprevir and amprenavir. It is not recommended to co-administer fosamprenavir/ritonavir and telaprevir.

(continued)

Table 3 Continued

Concomitant Drug Class: Drug Name	Effect on Concentration of INCIVEK or Concomitant Drug	Clinical Comment
lopinavir/ritonavir*	↑ telaprevir ↔ lopinavir	Concomitant administration of telaprevir and lopinavir/ritonavir resulted in reduced steady-state telaprevir exposure, while the steady-state exposure to lopinavir was not affected. It is not recommended to coadminister lopinavir/ritonavir and telaprevir.
HIV-ANTIVIRAL AGENTS: REVERSE TRANSCRIPTASE INHIBITORS		
efavirenz*	↑ telaprevir ↑ efavirenz	Concomitant administration of telaprevir and efavirenz resulted in reduced steady-state exposures to telaprevir and efavirenz.
tenofovir disoproxil fumarate*	↔ telaprevir ↓ tenofovir	Concomitant administration of telaprevir and tenofovir disoproxil fumarate resulted in increased tenofovir exposure. Increased clinical and laboratory monitoring is warranted. Tenofovir disoproxil fumarate should be discontinued in patients who develop tenofovir-associated toxicities.
HORMONAL CONTRACEPTIVES/ESTROGEN		
ethinyl estradiol* norethindrone	↑ ethinyl estradiol ↔ norethindrone	Exposure to ethinyl estradiol was decreased when co-administered with telaprevir. Two effective non-hormonal methods of contraception should be used during treatment with telaprevir. Patients using estrogens as hormone replacement therapy should be clinically monitored for signs of estrogen deficiency. Refer also to *Contraindications (4), Warnings and Precautions (5.1), Use in Specific Populations (8.1), and Patient Counseling Information (17.1)*.
IMMUNOSUPPRESSANTS		
cyclosporine*	↓ cyclosporine	Plasma concentrations of cyclosporine and tacrolimus are markedly increased when co-administered with
sirolimus	↓ sirolimus	telaprevir. Plasma concentration of sirolimus may be increased when co-administered with telaprevir, though

tacrolimus*	↓ tacrolimus	this has not been studied. Significant dose reductions and prolongation of the dosing interval of the immunosuppressant to achieve the desired blood levels should be anticipated. Close monitoring of the immunosuppressant blood levels and frequent assessments of renal function and immunosuppressant-related side effects are recommended when co-administered with telaprevir. Tacrolimus may prolong the QT interval. The use of telaprevir in organ transplant patients has not been studied.
INHALED BETA AGONIST		
salmeterol	↓ salmeterol	Concentrations of salmeterol may be increased when co-administered with telaprevir. Concurrent administration of salmeterol and telaprevir is not recommended. The combination may result in an increased risk of cardiovascular adverse events associated with salmeterol, including QT prolongation, palpitations, and sinus tachycardia.
NARCOTIC ANALGESIC		
methadone*	↑R-methadone	Concentrations of methadone were reduced when co-administered with telaprevir. No adjustment of methadone dose is required when initiating co-administration of telaprevir. However, clinical monitoring is recommended as the dose of methadone during maintenance therapy may need to be adjusted in some patients.
PDE5 INHIBITORS		
sildenafil	↓PDE5 inhibitors	Concentrations of PDE5 inhibitors may be increased when co-administered with telaprevir. For the treatment
tadalafil		of erectile dysfunction, sildenafil at a single dose not exceeding 25 mg in 48 hours, vardenafil at a single
vardenafil		dose not exceeding 2.5 mg dose in 72 hours, or tadalafil at a single dose not exceeding 10 mg dose in 72 hours can be used with increased monitoring for PDE5 inhibitor-associated adverse events. QT interval prolongation has been reported with vardenafil. Caution is warranted and clinical monitoring is recommended. Co-administration of sildenafil and telaprevir in the treatment of pulmonary arterial hypertension is contraindicated [see *Contraindications (4)*]. Co-administration of tadalafil and telaprevir in the treatment of pulmonary arterial hypertension is not recommended.

* These interactions have been studied. The direction of the arrow (↓ – increase, ↑ – decrease, ↔ – no change) indicates the direction of the change in PK.

Identification of Severity and Management of Rasha

The following guide includes examples and descriptions of mild, moderate, and severe rash that may occur during INCIVEK combination treatment.b

Mild rash 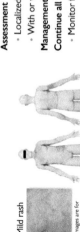 aImages are for illustrative purposes only	**Assessment** • Localized rash and/or a rash with limited distribution • With or without associated pruritus **Management** **Continue all drugs** • Monitor for signs of progression or development of systemic symptoms. • INCIVEK dose should not be reduced or interrupted. • Consider good skin care practices. • Consider oral antihistamines (sedating and/or non-sedatingc). • Consider topical corticosteroids (systemic corticosteroids are not recommended). **If progression or systemic symptoms are observed, reassess severity and proceed accordingly.**
Moderate rash 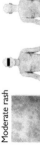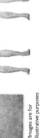 aImages are for illustrative purposes only	**Assessment** • Diffuse rash • With or without superficial skin peeling, pruritus, or mucous membrane involvement with no ulceration **Management** **Continue all drugs** • Monitor for signs of progression or development of systemic symptoms. • INCIVEK dose should not be reduced or interrupted. • Consider good skin care practices. • Consider oral antihistamines (sedating and/or non-sedatingc). • Consider topical corticosteroids (systemic corticosteroids are not recommended). **If progression or systemic symptoms are observed, reassess severity and proceed accordingly.**

Severe rash

*Images are for illustrative purposes only

Assessment

◦ Generalized rash with or without pruritus

OR

◦ Rash with vesicles, bullae, or ulcerations (other than SJS)

Management

Discontinue INCIVEK

May continue pegIFN-RBV

◦ Closely monitor for signs of progression.

◦ If rash does not improve within 7 days of INCIVEK discontinuation (or earlier if worsening rash), consider interruption or discontinuation of RBV and/or pegIFN.

◦ Earlier interruption or discontinuation of RBV and/or pegIFN-RBV may be needed if medically indicated.

◦ Consider utility of good skin care practices.

◦ Consider oral antihistamines (sedating and/or non-sedatingc).

◦ Consider topical corticosteroids (systemic corticosteroids are not recommended).

◦ INCIVEK must not be restarted after discontinuation.

◦ Consider dermatology consult.

Table 4 Drugs that Are Contraindicated with VICTRELIS

Drug Class	Drugs Within Class that Are Contraindicated with VICTRELIS	Clinical Comments
Alpha 1-Adrenoreceptor antagonist	Alfuzosin	Increased alfuzosin concentrations can result in hypotension.
Anticonvulsants t	Carbamazepine, phenobarbital, phenytoin	May lead to loss of virologic response to VICTRELIS
Antimycobacterial	Rifampin	May lead to loss of virologic response to VICTRELIS
Ergot derivatives	Dihydroergotamine, ergonovine, ergotamine, methylergonovine	Potential for acute ergot toxicity characterized by peripheral vasospasm and ischemia of the extremities and other tissues
GI motility agent	Cisapride	Potential for cardiac arrhythmias
Herbal products	St. John's Wort (*Hypericum perforatum*)	May lead to loss of virologic response to VICTRELIS
HMG-CoA reductase inhibitors	Lovastatin, simvastatin	Potential for myopathy, including rhabdomyolysis
Oral contraceptives	Drosperinone	Potential for hyperkalemia
PDE5 enzyme inhibitor	REVATIO® (sildenafil) or ADCIRCA® (tadalafil) when used for the treatment of pulmonary arterial hypertension*	Potential for PDE5 inhibitor-associated adverse events, including visual abnormalities, hypotension, prolonged erection, and syncope
Neuroleptic	Pimozide	Potential for cardiac arrhythmias
Sedative/hypnotics	Triazolam; orally administered midazolam†	Prolonged or increased sedation or respiratory depression

* See *Drug Interactions, Table 6* for coadministration of sildenafil and tadalafil when dosed for erectile dysfunction.

† See *Drug Interactions, Table 6* for parenterally administered midazolam.

Table 5

Adverse Events	Previously Untreated (SPRINT1 & SPRINT2)		Previous Treatment Failures (RESPOND2)	
	Percentage of Subjects Reporting Adverse Events		Percentage of Subjects Reporting Adverse Events	
Body System Organ Class	VICTRELIS + PegIntron + REBETOL (n=1,225)	PegIntron + REBETOL (n=467)	VICTRELIS + PegIntron + REBETOL (n=323)	PegIntron + REBETOL (n=80)
Median Exposure (days)	197	216	253	104
Blood and Lymphatic System Disorders				
Anemia	50	30	45	20
Neutropenia	25	19	14	10
Gastrointestinal Disorders				
Nausea	46	42	43	38
Dysgeusia	35	16	44	11
Diarrhea	25	22	24	16
Vomiting	20	13	15	8
Dry mouth	11	10	15	9
General Disorders and Administration Site Conditions				
Fatigue	58	59	55	50
Chills	34	29	33	30
Asthenia	15	18	21	16
Metabolism and Nutrition Disorders				
Decreased Appetite	25	24	26	16
Musculoskeletal and Connective Tissue Disorders				

(continued)

Table 5 Continued

Adverse Events	Previously Untreated (SPRINT1 & SPRINT2)		Previous Treatment Failures (RESPOND2)	
	Percentage of Subjects Reporting Adverse Events		Percentage of Subjects Reporting Adverse Events	
Body System Organ Class	VICTRELIS + PegIntron + REBETOL (n=1,225)	PegIntron + REBETOL (n=467)	VICTRELIS + PegIntron + REBETOL (n=323)	PegIntron + REBETOL (n=80)
Arthralgia	19	19	23	16
Nervous System Disorders				
Dizziness	19	16	16	10
Psychiatric Disorders				
Insomnia	34	34	30	24
Irritability	22	23	21	13
Respiratory, Thoracic, and Mediastinal Disorders				
Dyspnea (exertional)	8	8	11	5
Skin and Subcutaneous Tissue Disorders				
Alopecia	27	27	22	16
Dry Skin	18	18	22	9
Rash	17	19	16	6

Table 6 Established and Other Potentially Significant Drug Interactions

Concomitant Drug Class: Drug Name	Effect on Concentration of Boceprevir or Concomitant Drug	Recommendations
Endothelin receptor antagonist: bosentan	↑ bosentan	Concentrations of bosentan may be increased when co-administered with VICTRELIS. Use with caution and monitor closely.
HIV non-nucleoside reverse transcriptase inhibitors: efavirenz	↓ boceprevir*	Plasma trough concentrations of boceprevir were decreased when VICTRELIS was co-administered with efavirenz, which may result in loss of therapeutic effect. Avoid combination.
HIV protease inhibitors: ritonavir	↓ boceprevir* ↑ or ↓ HIV protease inhibitors	Boceprevir concentrations are decreased with ritonavir; the effect of ritonavir-boosted HIV protease inhibitors on boceprevir exposure is unknown. The effect of VICTRELIS on HIV protease inhibitor concentrations is unknown.
HMG-CoA reductase inhibitors: atorvastatin	↑ atorvastatin	Titrate atorvastatin dose carefully and do not exceed maximum daily dose of 20 mg during co-administration with VICTRELIS.
Immunosuppressants: cyclosporine, sirolimus, tacrolimus	↑immunosuppressants	Plasma concentrations of cyclosporine, sirolimus, and tacrolimus are expected to be increased significantly during co-administration with VICTRELIS. Close monitoring of immunosuppressant blood levels is recommended.
Inhaled beta-agonist: salmeterol	↑ salmeterol	Concurrent use of inhaled salmeterol and VICTRELIS is not recommended due to the risk of cardiovascular events associated with salmeterol.
Narcotic analgesic/opioid dependence: methadone, buprenorphine	↑ or ↓ methadone ↑ or ↓ buprenorphine	Plasma concentrations of methadone or buprenorphine may increase or decrease when co-administered with VICTRELIS. However, the combination has not been studied. Clinical monitoring is recommended as the dose of methadone or buprenorphine may need to be altered during concomitant treatment with VICTRELIS.

(continued)

Table 6 Continued

Concomitant Drug Class: Drug Name	Effect on Concentration of Boceprevir or Concomitant Drug	Recommendations
Oral hormonal contraceptives: drospirenone/ethinyl estradiol	↑ drospirenone* ↓ ethinyl estradiol*	The effect of boceprevir on other progestins is unknown; however, increases in exposure are anticipated. Concentrations of ethinyl estradiol are decreased in the presence of boceprevir. Systemic hormonal contraceptives should not be relied upon as an effective method of contraception in women during treatment with VICTRELIS. Two alternative effective methods of contraception should be used during combination treatment with ribavirin, and may include intrauterine devices and barrier methods [see Use in Specific Populations (8.1)].
PDE5 inhibitors: sildenafil, tadalafil, vardenafil	↑ sildenafil ↑ tadalafil ↑ vardenafil	Increases in PDE5 inhibitor concentrations are expected and may result in an increase in adverse events, including hypotension, syncope, visual disturbances, and priapism. Use of REVATIO® (sildenafil) or ADCIRCA® (tadalafil) for the treatment of pulmonary arterial hypertension (PAH) is contraindicated with VICTRELIS [see Contraindications (4)]. Use of PDE5 inhibitors for erectile dysfunction: Use with caution in combination with VICTRELIS, with increased monitoring for PDE5 inhibitor-associated adverse events. Do not exceed the following doses: Sildenafil: 25 mg every 48 hours; Tadalafil: 10 mg every 72 hours; Vardenafil: 2.5 mg every 24 hours.
Sedative/hypnotics: alprazolam; IV midazolam	↑ midazolam ↑ alprazolam	Close clinical monitoring for respiratory depression and/or prolonged sedation should be exercised during co-administration of VICTRELIS. A lower dose of IV

Antiarrhythmics: amiodarone, bepridil, flecainide, propafenone, quinidine	↑ antiarrhythmics	Co-administration with VICTRELIS has the potential to produce serious and/or life-threatening adverse events and has not been studied. Caution is warranted and therapeutic concentration monitoring of these drugs is recommended if they are used concomitantly with VICTRELIS.
digoxin	↑ digoxin	Digoxin concentrations may be increased with VICTRELIS. Use the lowest dose initially. with careful titration and monitoring of serum digoxin concentrations.
Anticoagulant: warfarin	↑ or ↓ warfarin	Concentrations of warfarin may be altered when coadministered with VICTRELIS. Monitor INR closely.
Antidepressants: trazodone,	↑ trazodone	Plasma concentrations of trazodone and desipramine
desipramine	↑ desipramine	may increase when administered with VICTRELIS,
		resulting in adverse events such as dizziness,
		Hypotension. and syncope. Use with caution and consider
		a lower dose of trazodone or desipramine.
Antifungals: ketoconazole,	↑ boceprevir*	Plasma concentrations of ketoconazole, itraconazole,
itraconazole, posaconazole,		voriconazole. or posaconazole may be increased with
voriconazole	↑ itraconazole ↑ ketoconazole ↑ posaconazole ↑ voriconazole	VICTRELIS. When co-administration is required, doses of ketoconazole and itraconazole should not exceed 200 mg/day.
Anti-gout: colchicine	↑ colchicine	Significant increases in colchicine levels are expected; fatal colchicine toxicity has been reported with other strong CYP3A4 inhibitors. Patients with renal or hepatic impairment should not be given colchicine with VICTRELIS. Treatment of gout flares (during treatment with VICTRELIS): 0.6 mg (1 tablet) x 1 dose, followed by 0.3 mg (half tablet) 1 hour later. Dose to be repeated no earlier than 3 days. Prophylaxis of gout flares (during treatment with VICTRELIS): If the original regimen was 0.6 mg twice a day, reduce dose to 0.3 mg once a day. If the original regimen was 0.6 mg once a day, reduce the dose to 0.3 mg once every other day. Treatment of familial Mediterranean fever (FMF) (during treatment with VICTRELIS): Maximum daily dose of 0.6 mg (maybe given as 0.3 mg twice a day).

(continued)

Table 6 Continued

Concomitant Drug Class: Drug Name	Effect on Concentration of Boceprevir or Concomitant Drug	Recommendations
Anti-infective: clarithromycin	↑ clarithromycin	Concentrations of clarithromycin may be increased with VICTRELIS; however, no dosage adjustment is necessary for patients with normal renal function.
Antimycobacterial:	↓ boceprevir	Increases in rifabutin exposure are anticipated, while
rifabutin	↑ rifabutin	exposure of boceprevir may be decreased. Doses have not been established for the two drugs when used in combination. Concomitant use is not recommended.
Calcium channel blockers, dihydropyridine: felodipine, nifedipine, nicardipine	↑ dihydropyridine calcium channel blockers	Plasma concentrations of dihydropyridine calcium channel blockers may increase when administered with VICTRELIS. Caution is warranted and clinical monitoring is recommended.
Corticosteroid, systemic: dexamethasone	↓ boceprevir	Co-administration of VICTRELIS with CYP3A4/5 inducers may decrease plasma concentrations of boceprevir, which may result in loss of therapeutic effect. Therefore, this combination should be avoided if possible and used with caution if necessary.
Corticosteroid, inhaled: budesonide, fluticasone	↑ budesonide ↑ fluticasone	Concomitant use of inhaled budesonide or fluticasone with VICTRELIS may result in increased plasma concentrations of budesonide or fluticasone, resulting in significantly reduced serum cortisol concentrations. Avoid co-administration if possible, particularly for extended duration.

Index